Nice and **F.A.T.**
(**F**ar **A**way from the **T**ruth)

Renita Brannan

&

Monica Hannan

Semper Distinguit Publications

Cover design by Studio Bickett

Editing and interior design by Cliff Naylor, Jr.

ISBN: 0-9984364-0-2
ISBN-13: 978-0-9984364-0-1

DEDICATION

This book is dedicated to anyone who has ever struggled with yo-yo dieting in an attempt to get healthy.

CONTENTS

Acknowledgments

Team work really does make the dream work. After two years of writing and editing, and yet more editing, we are beyond grateful that this book has become a reality. We earnestly believe it will be life-changing for all who read it.

Renita:

A special thank you to my husband, Scott, who tirelessly reworked our original draft to bring two incredible perspectives together. In addition, for the countless hours I spent writing and rewriting while he always kept our family rocking. He is a fantastic husband and father. To my boys, Beau, Truitt, and Rocco who have heard me say "PFC Every 3" at least 10,000 times and have sacrificed time with me so I can help change millions of lives with this message. They are living examples of what I teach and God has mighty plans for them! Remember boys, readers are leaders. Dream BIG, work hard, and expect great things!

To my dad, Richard Rhone, for helping me develop an incredible work ethic. To my beautiful mother, Pearl Rhone, for teaching me how to cook from scratch without measuring and make things taste great. But most importantly, for teaching me to never give up. "It will get better Nita," I have heard mom say on countless occasions.

To my friends and business partners, Stephanie Sandstrom and Mark Macdonald, who have dedicated as much passion and time to the cause of wellness as I have. I am so grateful for you both. Stephanie, you have been a Godsend to me in the past three years and I could not do what I do without your collaboration. Mark, you changed the course of my life five years ago when you taught me the message of PFC Every 3. I prayed for God to give me the secret to permanent weight loss, and He did just that, through you.

To my best friend, Jacinta Engelhardt, for leading me to Jesus Christ so I could understand the amazing plan God had for me. Because of you Jacinta, I realized my Kingdom assignment on Earth.

To Leota Neigum and all of my amazing clients and class participants over the last 20 years. You all INSPIRE me!!

To God, for giving me an incredible mission while on Earth. The best is yet to come!

Monica:

A special thank you to our book editor, Cliff Naylor, Jr., who thought of all the things we forgot. Who knew you'd turn out to be so detail oriented? You make me proud. To my girls, Meghanne and Hannah, who amaze me in so many ways, with their beauty, strength and honesty. When I look at you I see a bright future. And to my husband, partner, and friend, Cliff, who walks beside me on this incredible life journey. Thank you for your willingness to support and encourage me in a whole new way of living. I love you all. And finally, to Renita, who never once let me give up and who continues to be my inspiration day after day. You are one of life's great leaders.

Foreword

Imagine walking into a room and seeing an individual so passionate that every word she speaks inspires you to want to be better, live better and make your health truly matter. That's the experience I had back in January 2012, the day I first met Renita Brannan.

That day, Renita's energy was magnificent. Every word she said created a feeling of strength and determination and as each second ticked, you could feel the audience becoming more and more empowered to see the possibility of forever achieving their health goals.

I often think about that first encounter with Renita, and how special she is. Her heart, authenticity and shear desire to lead a real health change throughout society is as rare as the most precious diamond.

On that day, Renita, her husband Scott and their three incredible boys instantly became family. I met a kindred spirit, because just like Renita, for the last 20 years, my life's passion has been to help people stop dieting and start living their best health.

I've personally coached over 50,000 clients and helped millions of people make their health a priority. I wish this book had been published 20 years ago. Every one of my clients would have read it; but the good news is they now can!

Renita and Monica have written a masterpiece.

Nice and F.A.T. tells the real story behind losing weight, burning fat, increasing energy and most important, getting a real education about food and how to evolve that education into a way of life for you and your family.

This book takes you on a ride like you've never been on before. You'll see both sides to the challenges, limiting beliefs and massive breakthroughs we each experience during our health journey.

Monica shares her story in such a raw and honest way, and Renita provides the motivating support, nutrition facts and needed inspiration to help Monica push through and take her body and results to a place she never thought possible.

Nice and F.A.T. is much greater than a cutting edge nutrition and fitness book, it's the book everyone needs to read. It's the first book written in real time, focusing on the emotional obstacles we each face during our health journey and the impactful solutions to burst through those obstacles with powerful nutrition science.

I want to share with you one of my favorite quotes from the late Nelson Mandela: "True greatness is when you choose to exceed the expectations of yourself."

Make this the moment you draw your line in the sand and choose to exceed the expectations you have for your health.

This book is your vehicle to learning the tools to forever unlocking your body's full potential!

Get ready next level! Here you come....

-Mark Macdonald, *New York Times* bestselling author of *Body Confidence* and international health and fitness expert.

A Note to the Reader

There are three voices in this book:

Monica's in plain script,

Renita's in bold,

and *Scripture in italics.*

We also hope you'll take advantage of the journaling opportunities you'll find here. Studies have shown you're much more likely to meet your goals when you write them down.

Chapter 1
The Big F.A.T. Truth

Like you, I have my own story and life experience. I'm very excited to share with you parts of my journey, my results, and all I've learned. I'm thankful to be on this journey with you and thrilled to introduce my friend, Renita Brannan. Renita is a passionate health and fitness expert. She is committed to helping you live an abundantly healthy life. Renita believes your best days are ahead of you. I believe she will not only help you transform your body into a fat burning machine, but will empower you to enjoy the permanent results you want and the life you are longing for.

Through years of advanced education and experience, Renita has become an international health leader and life changer. She has been an important part of my health journey and together we are excited to partner with you.

So let's get real. There's something you want. It's going to take telling the truth and learning the truth for you to get it. I had to learn this myself. As a news anchor, my truth was I needed to make some positive changes. When she asked the question, "What do you want?" I told Renita I wanted to run a 5k. Really, though, I wanted to be skinny, or so I thought. But truthfully, I wanted so much more.

Most of us don't see ourselves aging all at once. We think we're going along fine and one day something compels us to *really* look in the mirror. In a glance, we wonder where that younger self went. For me, the mirror habit is an occupational hazard. If you manage to kid yourself on how your appearance actually is, the television viewer will usually offer a wake-up call. People actually call the station and send emails to say they don't like a reporter's style, or to say someone is fat or ugly. It happens. Those calls have always impacted me. Bigger than that was my personal wake-up call while looking at pictures from my son's wedding. I hated how I looked. Shortly afterward, we started our new show on NBC, *North Dakota Today*. This was my call to action.

Talk shows are a different animal in the television world. News people are allowed to be more formal. They can still wear blazers every day and I'd been hiding behind mine. The talk show format calls for a more casual, hip kind of look. In order to pull it off, I knew I had to get "hip" in a hurry. It's tougher to do if you can't fit into any of the cute styles that other talk show hosts are wearing. Have you noticed, for instance, that the women's dresses on daytime shows are almost always sleeveless? On the networks the co-hosts are not always young, but they do tend to be in great shape. These days it's less about age and more about tone, as in toned biceps. I had always wanted to do a talk show because they're a lot of fun and it was a new challenge for me, but for reasons already stated, I was worried. I needed the viewer to "see" me in the role of talk show host. It was time to make some drastic changes. I knew exercise was an important component in weight loss and overall fitness. I thought I could just ease into it. A daily walk, perhaps, or a step-aerobics class – those were my initial thoughts. So why in the world, out of nowhere, would I think of running a 5k?

My family and friends know I have always hated to run. As a

youngster I was actually pretty fast. Unfortunately, I had undiagnosed asthma and grew up associating running with pain and panic when my airway would start to close off, so I instinctively avoided it. Anybody who has asthma knows that it may produce fewer symptoms with age but it never really goes away. Mine would rear its ugly head if I was around cats, or if I had an upper respiratory infection, but a full blown attack was fairly rare. I wanted to keep it that way, so running was not something I'd even considered doing.

That's why it's so surprising that on the air one day I said to my co-host, Kevin Stanfield, "You know what? I think I'm going to run a 5K. I'm going to challenge myself." I really gave it very little thought beforehand.

Once I'd said it publically, though, I felt I was committed. The moment we got off the air I thought, "Oh no! What did I just do?" My first thought after that was, "I better call Renita!"

I didn't really know Renita well, having met her only a few times in the course of my work as a health reporter. I knew she'd been in the fitness field for more than a decade and that she had the kind of drive and personality that I could draw on. I asked Kevin to call her first, to see if she'd be willing to train me and come on the show as we made what I hoped would be progress. She immediately said yes.

Once the wheels were in motion I knew pride would not allow me to back out and besides, I'll do anything for a good story.

Let's start here. The first question I asked Monica is the first question I'll ask you. Tell me the truth. What is it that you really want?

I want:

What I will get from this:

_____

_____

POWER VERSE:

"And you will know the truth, and the truth will set you free." -John 8:32 NLT

Chapter 2
Sausage Fingers

After the initial phone call, Renita wasted no time getting in touch with me. She makes it her mission in life to get people healthy, and once she starts, look out! Here's the first thing she said to me: "Monica, before we start running we need to look at your health (she meant weight). It will be harder on your joints and lungs to run with this extra weight. Let's detox the bloat and inflammation before you begin. If you run 10 pounds lighter, it will be easier on every part of you, including your mind."

I remember thinking, "If detox means getting skinny, count me in." Who doesn't want to lose the bloat? That was certainly the case for me. I spent 20 years trying to lose the weight I gained with my second pregnancy. Like so many Americans (108 million people per year on average), I tried to whittle down the waistline by going on one diet plan after another. Particularly memorable was a diet I tried that involved nothing but cabbage soup the first day, nothing but bananas the second, and baked potatoes the third. At the end of day one, I felt as if I'd swallowed a helium balloon, not to mention the socially unacceptable consequences. I figured day two would be better as I love bananas. The diet said, "Eat as many as you want." I wanted a lot. Six hours later a severe reaction set in. First, I felt an itching sensation. Shortly thereafter my fingers swelled to the size of sausages. My lips swelled, my mouth itched and I broke out in hives from head to foot. Apparently you can overdo "one of nature's perfect fruits." I later found out that it's not unusual for people to react badly to a boatload of bananas. I started out on the diet fat. Now I was fat with a swollen tongue, body itches, hives and sausage fingers. Mercifully, I never got to the third day.

Most diets that people choose are restrictive. They force you to eliminate entire food groups, or they drastically restrict your calories while encouraging you to exercise. There are problems with that, as anybody who's ever been on a diet knows. Your first enemy is your own body. If you eat the same things day in and day out while eliminating all of the foods that nature intended for us to enjoy, you'll develop cravings that will become difficult, if not impossible, to ignore. Eventually, you'll give in.

And if you restrict your calories you may lose weight at first, until your body realizes you're starving it. Once it catches on, it goes into what we in the television industry refer to as "slow-mo." Restrict your calories enough and before long it won't matter how much exercise you do, you're going to have trouble losing weight. The end result is discouragement, and there you are again, attached to that yo-yo string.

The truth is, there are some crazy diets out there.

What's the craziest diet you've ever been on?

_____

_____

How did you feel when you were on this diet?

_____

_____

What did you learn?

_____

_____

If we are going to embrace the journey we have to stop feeling guilty about past failures. As we move through this book, we may stop to identify exactly what happened. How did it make us feel? What did we learn?

It is what it is. Like Monica's banana diet, maybe there is humor in it. Laugh a little! Joy does the body good.

POWER VERSE:

"So whether you eat or drink or whatever you do, do it all for the glory of God." -1 Corinthians 10:31 NIV

Chapter 3
Shake Your Groove Thing

Wake up! Forget what you've learned about dieting! It has failed you and if you are willing to grow, you will never diet again! You are about to lay down a brand new groove in your brain, understanding how to nourish your body with food. We must get out of the old ruts that have not led us to victory. The ruts in our brains, the ruts in our habits, and the ruts in our attitudes.

When I began this journey I didn't know the truth, but I know it now. The truth is diets usually don't work. As evidence, the weight loss industry is booming to the tune of $300 billion annually. Stop and think about it. If people were really having success, the numbers would be declining rather than increasing. Many people fall off the weight-go-round chasing a skinny body. The truth is, for most people the long term results never happen. In fact, many times we actually "sell out" to short term results at the expense of our health.

To get healthy and stay that way, I've discovered you simply cannot starve yourself or eat nothing but cabbage soup followed by bananas. The last thing you should do is cut out fat or stop eating carbs. The truth is, food is not the enemy, nor is it the friend that makes all things better.

We should enjoy the taste of food, but also enjoy and understand how food nourishes our bodies, energizes us, and gives us life. It's the unhealthy emotional connection to food that can lead us down the wrong path. Food should be our greatest ally in healthy weight-loss and feeling our absolute best. Now that we're on this incredible new journey together, we will learn that food is vital to a healthy life. It's an essential fuel. As we learn to reshape the way we think about food, our lives will be changed forever.

The truth is we all want to create better habits.

Currently, you probably crave certain foods that make you feel like hell. Shortly after eating these foods you feel guilty, tired, ashamed, lethargic, weak, and foggy.

Tell yourself, I'm ready to "let go" of these foods today:

_____

_____

The truth is you are capable of creating better habits. Right now, think of foods that make you feel nourished, happy, energized, free of guilt, and full of life.

I am ready to embrace these foods today:

_____

_____

If you have no idea what these foods are don't worry! Read on...YOU ARE ABOUT TO LEARN!

POWER VERSE:

"Do not conform to the pattern of this world, but be transformed by the renewing of your mind. Then you will be able to test and approve what God's will is - His good, pleasing and perfect will." - Romans 12:2 NIV

Chapter 4
Stinky Fish

What memories and imprints helped create your beliefs regarding food? Many times our likes and dislikes regarding food can be traced back to an emotional experience, either bad or good.

This self-reflection is an important step to getting healthy. My earliest memory involves a contest of wills between my mother and her mother-in-law, my grandmother. We were at a family gathering and my mother, no doubt needing a break from the chaos that large families create, was fixing me a bottle to take to bed with me. For years my mother would tell people that I had a bottle until I was old enough to fix it myself, and it was true. My grandmother was appalled, but I can understand why my mother did it. She was barely out of her teens herself and had given birth to two children in under a year, my older brother born in May, and me the following April. At the end of the day she simply needed a break and a little time to herself.

This was in the early 60s, a time when a typical father's family involvement was to bring home a paycheck, toss the ball in the backyard and offer guidance a la Ward Cleaver. My father changed exactly one diaper while my brother and I were babies.

Once, my mother went out to a ladies event and left us napping. While she was gone I had a messy diaper that couldn't be ignored. She tells me how she came home to find me dry, but with the diaper bunched up in front with a single safety pin holding it together. It was more like a crisis intervention.

Contrary to this, my husband was involved in every aspect of our children's early years, from walking the floor at night with a fussy infant to giving them their baths. Even though my mother's situation and mine are not exactly the same, now that I'm the mother of three I get it.

I don't know if those bedtime bottles were the start of my nightly bedtime ritual, but I never carried a blanket, I didn't suck my thumb, and I didn't have a favorite stuffed animal. For me it was all about the food.

Here's an example of my diet in first grade. When my mother worked, breakfast was a bowl of cereal, sometimes hot although I didn't really enjoy that over Captain Crunch or Lucky Charms. For lunch it was a bologna sandwich on white bread with mayo, a bag of chips, a Scooter Pie, and an apple which I always threw away. The school provided a carton of whole milk. There was usually an after-school snack consisting of cookies and more milk, or cake and milk. Kool-Aid was always readily available too. If I fell and hurt myself, my mother soothed me with food. The remedy for a bad day at school was hot chocolate and cookies.

My mother was and still is a great cook. But most of the information we have now regarding health wasn't readily available or applied in the 1960s. Plus, there were years when money was tight. Growing up, I could count on the same basic meal nearly every night. There was a starch, canned vegetable, iceberg lettuce salad and a piece of meat. One night might be hamburger patties with ketchup, boiled potatoes with butter, lettuce with oil and vinegar, and canned string beans. The next night it was fried chicken with Minute Rice and corn. A third night might be pork chops with fried potatoes and apple sauce. Throw in the occasional spaghetti with meat sauce and garlic toast, a hot dish or two and steaks on the grill with fries on the side and you've got the average American diet of the 60s and 70s. Oh, and there was one night a week when my mother cooked liver and onions, because "it's good for you." I hated it, but she always fried it in bacon grease. The reward for eating the liver was the bacon. And the reward for eating it all was chocolate cake or lemon meringue pie for dessert.

Fast food was a rarity. Occasionally my parents would take us out to dinner, where the main course was always beef for me, usually a big, fat hamburger. Living where we did in California's Napa Valley, we made the occasional trip to Fisherman's Wharf. I always associated seafood with the smell of the wharf and refused to eat fish. My mother didn't really care for it either, so there was never an argument. What I did like, though, were deep fried prawns in sweet and sour sauce on the nights we had Chinese takeout, and on occasion my father would bring home sourdough bread and hard salami, which we ate in lieu of supper.

Whatever the meal laid before me, like many of you I'm sure, if I finished everything on my plate I was applauded and nearly always rewarded with dessert. I was a proud member of the "Clean Plate Club."

It's probably not surprising that as I got older my parents both began to have a weight problem. My mother was built like a '50s pin-up girl, but as we grew up and her activity level decreased, she, too, began to see the pounds add up. It didn't help that at around the time I started junior high my father was transferred to North Dakota. The cold climate was a real shock to Mom, being a California girl through and through. Dad traveled for his work and she frequently found herself alone with not much to do. She turned to comfort eating, and comfort cooking. My favorite time of the week was Saturday morning because she'd take me grocery shopping with her and we'd fill the cart with snack foods I loved, along with the good foods that she planned to prepare for supper.

One of the ways my amazing mother showed her love was to feed us, but in our childhood years, she lacked the nutritional foundation and understanding of how to stabilize our blood sugar and prepare properly balanced meals and snacks.

Reflecting on "food memories" was a great exercise for me. I discovered how and when I developed unhealthy associations with food. I realized that I was given food for comfort and rewards, and that it equaled love for me.

The truth is past events lay the foundation for our existing views of food. These events created a belief in Monica and started a pattern in her life. Does your foundation need a massive uprooting and renovation?

It doesn't mean you're not thankful for the good people and good things in your life.

If you're going to lose weight and be healthy, it's important for you to tell the truth about how and why you see food the way you do.

What are some "food memories" you have growing up?

_____

_____

How did this make you feel?

_____

_____

What did you learn?

_____

_____

You must create healthy new thoughts and beliefs about food in order to lose weight and be healthy.

We will help you!

POWER VERSE:

"You were taught with regard to your former way of life, to put off your old self, which is being corrupted by its deceitful desires; to be made new in the attitude of your minds; and to put on a new self, created to be like God in true righteousness and holiness." -Ephesians 4:22-24 NIV

Chapter 5
Sweet Rolls and Sore Throats

A crappy diet doesn't always make you fat, but believe me, you'll feel crappy.

As I entered my teen years, I started to identify with ill health instead of aligning myself with the truth. Again looking back, when boredom finally got the better of my mother she rejoined the workforce and there was a shift in lifestyle for all of us. My dad's travels meant he was typically home only on the weekend. My mother didn't want to drive in the snow so she didn't apply for a North Dakota driver's license, which meant she had to walk to and from work, a roundtrip of several miles. Back then most kids walked to and from school as well. That forced regular exercise on all of us. Plus, she had less time to cook, so there was less of an emphasis on baked goods. She worked in a clinic that specialized in heart disease and she could clearly see the effects of a good old home-cooked meal. We still got the same basic foods at home, but she tried to incorporate more fresh vegetables, she grew a garden and there was more of an emphasis on plain meats, well cooked, and less of an emphasis on gravy. Unfortunately for me, the die was already cast. I was already addicted to sugar and was at an age where there was less parental control over my diet.

I was luckier than most in that unlike my parents, my body type was more what you'd call "sturdy," rather than fat. I was athletically built with narrow hips and broad shoulders, and I didn't tend to pack on pounds when I was younger. I wasn't skinny, mind you, but I never got fat either. The upside was that I didn't have to worry about my weight. The downside was that I could put whatever junk into my body I wanted and it didn't seem to have an outward effect – not at first, anyway.

By the time I was in high school I typically skipped breakfast at home altogether. At my school I could get a huge sweet roll mid-morning, which I usually did, washing it down with a can of Coke. For lunch it was almost always a choice of pizza, hamburgers or tacos, which I loved, and milk. I was still throwing that apple away. Dessert was a huge cookie. Mid-afternoon I would visit the candy store on campus and buy chocolate or suckers. One of my favorites was the Jolly Rancher, which we were allowed to eat during class. After school, before heading to tennis practice I'd grab a handful of cookies, now store-bought, and after a particularly hard match, I'd head straight for the convenience store and buy a can of Orange Crush. Did I feel good? No, not particularly. I had frequent colds, asthma at night, bladder infections, sinus infections and in one memorable case, trench mouth, but nobody ever said to me, "Gee, maybe it's your diet."

On My Own

When I got to college it got even worse. I didn't live in university housing, but in an apartment off campus. However, like most college students, funds were tight. My diet was pretty much the same, day in and day out. For breakfast it was six butter cookies from the Quality Bakery in Fargo and a Tab. For lunch I would sneak into the teachers' lounge on campus where there was always a pot of chili cooking. You could get a bowl of that and a carton of milk for 75 cents. I worked at the *The Forum of Fargo-Moorhead* newspaper in the evenings and supper was always a sandwich out of the vending machine and another Tab or two.

The only variable was when I had a sore throat, a frequent occurrence. At those times, I would sip on salty chicken bouillon, one of the options available in the machine that provided coffee, tea and hot chocolate. Sometimes I couldn't even afford to do that, so I'd head over to the Trader and Trapper lounge in Moorhead, just across the bridge from Fargo and just over the Minnesota line, where the drinking age was 19. It wasn't the alcohol that lured me. Rather, it was the pot of cheese spread and basket of crackers that they put on the tables. I'd order another Tab and sit there for an hour drinking that and eating the crackers until the cheese was gone. Before bed, no matter how broke I was, I always ate something rich and sweet, like donuts. Essentially, I was still putting myself to bed with that bottle.

By my third year at the university, that frequent sore throat became a constant, so much so that I became used to it and just ignored it. For some reason it never occurred to me to go to the campus clinic and get it checked out. I was hell bent on graduating in three years instead of the usual four, so my course load was heavy. With school and work I had little time for anything else, sleep included. As I neared the end of my college career I made arrangements to finish my last quarter of school as an intern at KFYR-TV in Bismarck, where my parents still lived. I showed up day after day not really feeling too peppy and with an asthmatic cough. It was the asthma that finally got me to the doctor. I woke up terrified one morning because I was unable to take a deep breath.

After a whole battery of tests, not only was the asthma pinpointed and finally treated, but something else showed up. It turned out that the sore throat and the general rundown feeling I'd had for many months was mononucleosis. I had gotten so used to running on empty that I didn't note it as being an unusual feeling.

The truth is... you get to choose. You MUST be intentional. If you are living on "autopilot" or "cruise control," the

foundational beliefs you developed in your youth will ultimately dictate how you see yourself.

Through a self-reflection process, Monica discovered how her foundational imprints developed into unhealthy habits, which led to actually identifying as a person of ill-health. Feeling sick was just "who she was." It was normal.

The more Monica learned, the more she started to see the relationship between eating in an unhealthy way and sickness. Monica chose what she ate. She chose her daily activities.

Monica used to say things like:

"I don't eat breakfast."

"I love junk food and diet soda."

"I can't afford to eat healthy."

"I used to be able to eat anything I wanted."

"I get sick all the time."

"I don't eat fish."

What are you currently saying about yourself?

_____

_____

Do these F.A.T. (Far Away from Truth) belief statements make you feel like a victim or an over-comer?

_____

_____

Why?

_____

_____

Are these F.A.T. (Far Away from Truth) identities keeping you from reaching your weight loss goals?

_____

_____

The truth is, you were created to be abundantly healthy- full of energy and vitality. You are not a victim. You are an over comer! You were designed in the image and likeness of the greatest champion who ever lived!

POWER VERSE:

"For as he thinks in his heart, so is he." -Proverbs 23:7 NKJV

Chapter 6
Loving Cliff and Diet Coke

Your body is made up of about 70% water. Diet Coke is not water. Water purifies our bodies inside and out. Would you ever clean the outside of your body by bathing in Diet Coke? Sounds like a sticky mess to me.

My first job in television happened by accident. That internship that I'd snagged ended up being in Williston, ND, where they were short-handed. I spent three months there, intending to go back to the *Forum* when I finished, but when the three months were up they hired me full-time. I only spent about eight months in Williston, but those months changed my life. The television station itself was an isolated place, located 13 miles out of town on a highway heading toward Montana. My job there was to report on anything that was happening around town and anchor the noon news. Winter that year was one of the worst on record and it came early.

When you work in a station that small, you have to learn to do everything yourself. These days the "one-man-band reporter" is the norm, as camera equipment has gotten smaller and lighter and easier to use. Back then, though, it was more unusual. I arrived in Williston without the slightest notion of how to shoot a news story. There was a photographer on staff at the time who shot commercials. He was auburn haired with a fiery red beard and what I thought was the temperament to go with it. I didn't know him at all, but he always walked around with an intense scowl on his face, and to be honest, I was a little afraid of him. Somebody higher up gave him the job of teaching me how to run the camera.

We went out on a frigidly cold day in early December for our first lesson and while he instructed me on the camera's intricacies, he kept glancing at my feet. The shoes I was wearing were more about fashion than practicality, and he finally said, "You have to be freezing in those things." It was an astute observation, because I was literally freezing my toes off, along with my fingers and my face. The temperature was hovering right around zero. He continued talking about how to shoot a news story but I had stopped listening. I was too busy shivering. He finally said, "Okay, that's it. Get in the car."

When I did, he turned the heater on full blast and said, "Look, I have to go let my dog out anyway, so we're going to my place and you're going to warm up." From that point on, Cliff Naylor and I were inseparable. He showed me how to shoot that winter, taught me how to play racquetball (poorly), went looking for me during a blizzard when I overshot the driveway of the station in the blinding snow, and finally bought me not one, but three pairs of mittens. In exchange, I gave him the mono that I'd been carrying for many months and nearly killed him, but that's another story. The bottom line is that after I met Cliff, my life improved dramatically.

Our next stop after Williston was a slightly bigger television station in Twin Falls, Idaho. Cliff chose that place specifically for its more moderate weather along with its close proximity to the mountains, and I was excited to go along. He was hired as a photographer but we hadn't been there long when he was promoted to evening sportscaster. I started out as a reporter but quickly moved into the anchor chair. On weekends we explored our surroundings and I got a chance to try new things like rock climbing in the Sawtooth Mountains, camping in the wilderness, and white water rafting. There was always something new to do and somewhere interesting to explore, and we also made great friends.

It was also about this time that I developed my love affair with Diet Coke. That probably doesn't seem like such a bad thing, having the occasional soft drink. But in my case it was an addiction. I had to have it first thing upon waking up in the morning and as the day went on I'd easily drink a six pack. I'd have a can on the nightstand so that if I woke up at night I could take a swig. I used that in place of water. Back then nobody really knew the effects of the sweetener aspartame and how harmful it is to our bodies. Because of the unknown effects, I gave it up completely during my pregnancies, but I craved it constantly. In fact, I was in the delivery room right after giving birth and they asked me if I needed anything and Diet Coke is what I asked for. I drank two cans before I even got down from the table.

I was hooked. I dreamed about Diet Coke. I tried to give it up on occasion but suffered frequent headaches and treated them with ibuprofen on a daily basis. For years, it wasn't unusual for me to take six or eight Advil in a day. I can't tell you if it was the aspartame, the caffeine, or something else altogether that caused them. But I do know that after 30 years of constant diet soda, I gave it up cold turkey one year for Lent. My headaches went away and I don't miss them one bit!

The truth is our faith in God, along with a gratitude-based perspective, can help us overcome our food addictions.

Monica made a commitment during Lent, a time when Catholics remember the incredible sacrifice Jesus made by suffering and dying on the cross for our sins. Now there's a champion role model! His love conquered sin and death! Can you imagine the torture and pain Jesus endured for us?

Diet Coke had a strong hold on Monica. But compared to the sacrifices Jesus made, giving up Diet Coke seemed small. This perspective and her faith commitment held her accountable. Forty days later, Diet Coke and the associated headaches were gone from her life.

These vices can start out small and build to have more power over us than we ever imagined they could.

What's that "one thing" you know you should give up?

_____

_____

What healthy alternative can you replace it with?

_____

_____

POWER VERSE:

"The temptations in your life are no different from what others experience. And God is faithful. He will not allow the temptation to be more than you can stand. When you are tempted, he will show you a way out so that you can endure." -1 Corinthians 10:13 NLT

Chapter 7
Baby Weight

As new parents, you will get fitter or fatter. The choice is ultimately yours to make. I suggest fitter! You don't get less busy with kids, you get more busy! Find a way to live as a healthy, active family! Little eyes and ears are always watching! Be a great role model! Loving and nourishing yourself is a great example to set for your children.

When God gifts us with children, it's our job to take care of them, and I believe most new parents do everything they can to ensure their children's health. Why is it, then, that we don't view our own health as the gift it is, and safeguard it in the same way?

When our first daughter, Meghanne, was born, Cliff and I were ridiculous. Like new parents everywhere, we were totally in love with her and made sure everybody knew it. We were still active, but now we had a constant sidekick with us, one who had to eat sensibly. Before she was born, as busy and young career-minded people, our mealtime was typically on-the-fly, but afterward we made sure there was a decent dinner on the table every night. Cliff did most of the cooking back then. I worked late at the television station, which often meant I'd eat a regular dinner that he had prepared, and when I got home after the late show, hungry again, I'd fix myself a snack, which, you guessed it, was something on the order of cookies, cake, pie, or ice cream.

One child is portable. Two children is a little more complicated. By the end of 1988 we were back in Bismarck, once again working at KFYR-TV, and our son C.J. was on the way. Once he was born it was more of a challenge to be active. That challenge was compounded by the birth of our third daughter, Hannah, and because North Dakota winters are so cold, we all too often used that as an excuse to stay indoors and park ourselves in front of the TV. It's not something we encouraged the children to do. In fact, we didn't have cable in our home until just a few years ago because we didn't want them sitting in front of a screen all day. We'd do family things until the kids' bedtime; reading stories, playing games, doing homework and supervising bath time. After that, though, the two of us watched movies while we munched on a big bowl of popcorn, followed up by a big bag of chocolate covered peanuts. We did encourage the kids to be involved in sports. Meg played tennis, C.J. played hockey, Hannah volleyball, and all three played soccer. But somewhere along the line I realized that I was passing along some of the same food habits that I'd grown up with. If they finished their meals they got a treat. Cliff's family had a tradition that we picked up, called their bedtime "party," which involved a sugary snack more often than not. I found myself comforting them with food as my mother did with me, and Cliff started doing it too.

My oldest daughter married in 2011 and we gathered for the traditional family pictures. As I was gazing at the proofs I saw something that I hadn't noticed before. My arms were getting heavy. And not just my arms, I had a spare tire around my middle that had crept up on me and I hadn't really noticed. That very week I bought a bathroom scale and for the first time in years started weighing myself. I was shocked at what the scale said. That's when I started dieting in earnest. I tried one plan after another. All of them worked for a short time but I couldn't imagine staying on any of them for the rest of my life. Within months I'd be back to eating the way I always had and I'd end up gaining all the weight back, and then some. This was a cycle that went on for a couple of years until 2013, when my son got married. Once again there were the family pictures, and once again I was shocked by what I saw. I had contented myself with the idea that it wasn't really so bad. I was no spring chicken, after all. Friends told me it's impossible after a certain point to take the weight off the middle. One told me that fat in the face contributes to a youthful appearance because it fills out the wrinkles. I latched onto those notions and bought looser clothes, trying to hide what I couldn't seem to control. But looking at the pictures this time I couldn't deny what I was seeing. I now felt fat and it was time to do something about it, because I wasn't feeling loving toward my body.

What parts of your body are you uncomfortable with?

Are you ready to love how you look and feel?

Are you ready to be an excellent role model for your children and grandchildren?

POWER VERSE:

"Do everything in love." -1 Corinthians 16:14 NIV

Chapter 8
Shake, Rattle, Roll...and Yo-Yo

Cutting calories is an outdated means of losing weight. It will always leave us hangry (hungry/angry) and fatter when the diet is over. Our bodies don't function on math, our bodies function on biology.

Despite the fact that I was slowly, year-by-year, putting on weight, I was still pretty active, or I thought I was. I played tennis once or twice a week and in the summer I liked to golf. But as for an organized exercise plan, forget it! I always thought that was boring, and I like to move, even if it's just to jiggle my restless legs. I did try yoga once. I went out and bought the mat and the cute little outfits. It was all about the fashion statement, as I recall. That was in the late 80s when we were all rocking the headbands and leg warmers. I got to class and was able to pretzel myself into the first couple of moves. I remember thinking to myself, what *is* this? Yoga was hard! Maybe instead of this, I should go find one of those exercise fat shakers (you know the kind I mean), where you just sort of stand there and the weight jiggles itself off while I read *War and Peace*. That was *my* kind of exercise plan. Or so I thought.

Most diet plans stress physical movement as an important

component to permanent weight loss. I can't argue with that. Every January the gyms are crowded with people who start out with the best of intentions. Surveys post weight loss as the top New Year's resolution. In the number two spot is a vow to exercise more. They naturally go together.

So let me ask you:

What was your New Year's Resolution last January 1st?

_____

_____

Did it create lasting results?

_____

_____

Let's face it, getting up and going to the gym every day is hard work. We all have 24 hours in a day. We all have choices to make each day. Exercise may be the last thing you want to do. If you don't make the right choices you will gain back the weight you lose, and more. Maybe you made resolutions to exercise and lose weight but it just didn't happen. Maybe by the end of the year you've actually gained weight and slowed your metabolism down through unhealthy and restrictive diets. Calorie counting doesn't work. Every deficit needs to be repaid. Maybe, you wasted money on another annual membership or bought an expensive piece of equipment (let's use Monica's term, the fat shaker) to hang your laundry on. Maybe you feel a little defeated, fat, and frustrated.

The insane cycle of lose, gain, and gain more shows up each year all over again, regardless of your New Year's resolution. There's a reason it's referred to as yo-yo dieting.

Today let's have courage and declare together, "I am ready to cut the diet yo-yo string!"

Because the truth is, diets don't work for permanent weight loss and health.

Are you ready to apply what Monica has learned? Are you ready for freedom? Are you ready to permanently turn on your metabolism?

Are you ready to never diet again? Let's get started!

POWER VERSE:

"Dear friend, I pray that you are doing well in every way. I pray that your body is strong and well even as your soul is." -3 John 2 NLV

Chapter 9
Excuses are Like...

My grandmother was the daughter of a homesteader in Burke, South Dakota, in 1913. She was the last of four daughters born to Cordelia and Joe Byrne at a time when life was hard and hard work was the norm. Just getting supper on the table was an all-day affair. Childhood was short. My grandmother once told me a story that brought this home. She said she wasn't very old when her parents left her home alone for the day with instructions that she was to prepare a roasted chicken for the family's supper that night. What that meant was going into the yard, selecting a chicken, killing it, plucking it, boiling it to remove the pin feathers, stuffing it, then stoking the coal-fired stove and roasting it. "I'd seen it done," she told me, "but I'd never tried to do it myself."

First she ran around the yard trying to catch the chicken but she couldn't get close enough to get her hands around its neck. Plus, she admitted that she was afraid of the bird, since chickens peck and scratch. Finally, after an hour of chasing and at the point of exhaustion, she went into the garden shed and found a pair of long-handled shears which she used to hack at the bird until it finally just gave up and died. It's clear my grandmother was not in need of an exercise program.

Life today, though, involves a lot of sitting for most of us. We're busy enough, from morning until we drop into bed at night, but we don't typically have to work as hard physically as they did in my grandmother's time. Consider laundry day. We complain if the machine isn't on the same floor as the dirty clothes. But for Grandma the chore involved pumping water into a tub, heating it on that same coal-burning stove, hauling the water and the clothes out to the porch, chopping soap into the water, scrubbing the clothes on a washboard, wringing them out and finally, hanging them on a clothesline to dry. It was an all-day, exhausting affair. Imagine the upper body workout it offered. My grandmother was born at the dawn of a new era in world history when life was about to become exponentially easier, but it would be a while before the Dakotas saw all of the benefits. Just as electricity was spreading to rural areas, World War II derailed fundraising efforts and rural families had to wait. When electric power finally did reach Burke, daily practices that had stayed the same for hundreds of years changed rapidly. With power to pump water, indoor plumbing became possible. Lamps no longer had to be'carried from room to room, and think what a difference refrigeration made, not to mention an electric stove or a vacuum cleaner. What also followed was a steady rise in obesity rates in the United States.

Prior to World War I, it was rare to see people who were seriously overweight. They worked too hard, and food was too time-consuming to prepare for people to "graze." In fewer than 100 years we've seen labor-saving technologies advance to the point where some people actually have robots to do their housework.

Other changes that have contributed to our expanding waistlines include the rise in processed foods, the advent of the fast-food culture as women joined the workforce, the prevalence of the automobile, the invention of radio and then television, and finally internet technology. I wouldn't give any of it up. I'm using all of those technologies right now, writing this book. But all one has to do is walk around the local Walmart to see what all of that sitting around is doing to the American butt. Two out of three in the U.S. are considered overweight. One in three is obese. For the first time in American history, our life expectancy is actually on the decline. We all want to do something about it, or at least we talk about doing something about it. It doesn't take long for the latest diet idea to reach fad status. New books on weight loss tend to skyrocket onto the best seller lists. Sometimes reading them is as far as we get. Or, like me with the cabbage soup diet, we start out on them, lose weight rapidly, go back to our regular lifestyle and end up gaining it all back plus a little more.

There are a lot of reasons why diets don't work for us. You probably recognize things you tell yourself on this list of the top ten reasons people give for their inability to either start or stick with a healthy lifestyle plan:

1. **I don't have time.**
2. **The diet is too restrictive.**
3. **I don't have self-control.**
4. **Healthy foods are too expensive.**
5. **I can't or don't like to cook.**
6. **I don't like cooking just for myself.**
7. **My family won't eat it.**
8. **Exercise is boring.**
9. **I'm too out of shape and it's too hard.**
10. **I've always focused on my weight rather than my health.**

Nothing great in life is achieved without identifying obstacles and committing yourself to overcoming them.

Which of these roadblocks can you relate to the most?

Are you willing to commit and utilize faith and courage to overcome what's standing between you and your goals?

_____

_____

POWER VERSE:

"The thief comes to steal, kill, and destroy; I have come that they may have life and have it to the full." -John 10:10

Chapter 10
I Don't Have Time

Monica voiced every one of those 10 excuses. It didn't take long for me to shoot them down, starting with her number one excuse, "I don't have time!"

Think about how crazy it sounds to say "I don't have time to be healthy." My question is, "What do you have time for?" For most of us, the "not enough time" excuse simply isn't true; it's a matter of setting priorities. Do you have time to spend on Facebook? Do you have time to watch *The Voice*? Do you have time for retail therapy? Change the way you think to: How can I work physical activity into this thing I love to spend my time doing? A great use of time would be to jump on a mini trampoline while you watch TV.

When I thought about it, I had to admit Renita was right. Let's start with food. One hundred years ago most of a woman's time was spent preparing meals. Like my grandmother, she often had to catch the meat before cooking it. She had to grow the vegetables and can the excess produce so she'd have it available when fresh food wasn't an option. Everything she made, she made from scratch. Consider the lowly flapjack. My grandmother likely had store-bought flour on hand, but she had to gather the eggs herself, which meant caring for the chickens, and she had to get the milk by milking a cow which also had to be fed and housed. The butter for the flapjacks had to be churned, the lard rendered from the pig that the family raised all year and then butchered in the fall. You get the idea. When you think of all that it probably does sound easier to drive down the street and buy an Egg McMuffin, but if you're honest with yourself as I have finally forced myself to be, you'd admit it takes just minutes to make blueberry pancakes if you have the ingredients on hand. You can even freeze them and let the kids microwave them when they're hungry. That roast chicken that my grandmother spent so much energy on can go from the fridge to your oven in the time it takes to unwrap the packaging and sprinkle on spices. If you're really strapped for time you can scrub some potatoes and bake them at the same time and eat them skins and all, which in the end is better for you. Or you can buy a chicken already cut up and throw it into the Crock-Pot with some barbecue sauce and set the timer for the minute you get home. Add a salad and some brown rice and you've got supper. What that takes is planning, which we'll talk more about later.

Now to the exercise we know we need, but think we don't have time for. It took about two months before I noticed a mind shift, and one day realized my pedometer had become my new best friend. These come in all varieties and in every price range. Some simply monitor the steps you take. Others actually nag you to get up and move when you've been sitting too long. Once you're wearing one you become much more aware of how much you move throughout your day. If you have a goal of 10,000 steps a day you'll find yourself parking on the fourth floor of the ramp just so you can take the four flights of steps down. You'll view your house or yard work as exercise opportunities because you know that at the end of the day, if you're only at 8,000 steps you'll need to hit the treadmill or run in place to hit your goal. Much better to get it while doing something constructive and/or enjoyable. And if your kids are your excuse, consider your own exercise as part of your parenting by example. They do what you do, so when you take them to soccer practice, make sure they see you walking up and down the sidelines. When you spend time with them, make it something active. Little kids are born loving to run and jump. If you keep them doing it, they'll continue to love it. Somewhere along the line, too many of us allow screens to take over our children's lives, setting them up for a lifetime of weight problems.

"I don't have time" may be the excuse I hear the most often. We all have seven days in a week and 24 hours in a day. It is common for most people to work for eight, sleep for eight, and then we *all* have the same eight hours to live life! Why is it that some people who are extremely busy and successful make time for a 30-minute workout while other people who sit on social media for two hours every day don't? It comes down to priorities. It is not as much a "time issue" as it is a "priority issue."

When you make time for your health, you will get healthier. I can't make the decision for you. It is not going to miraculously happen. We must plan, prepare, and equip ourselves for success. We have to live in these bodies for our entire lives, so it's time we make it a priority to be well.

Where can you find time in your day to take charge of your health? Be specific.

_____

_____

POWER VERSE:

"And do this, understanding the present time: the hour has already come for you to wake up from your slumber, because our salvation is nearer now than when we first believed. The night is nearly over; the day is almost here." -Romans 13:11-14

Chapter 11
This Diet is Too Restrictive

Many people say, "I don't want to restrict myself." If you are dieting, you are certainly doing that. I am a believer in nourishing your body. In fact, my goal is to help 100 million people take control of their health by ditching the diet mentality. YOU are one of them!

Here's where I had to learn to change my viewpoint from dieting to simply eating foods that are healthy. The popular term these days is "clean eating." Foods that are as close as possible to the way God made them. It's easier than ever to eat healthy because our choices are so vast and the food is, in many cases, ready to eat or fast to fix. Think about what you eat in a week. If you're like me, you reach for your favorites again and again, whatever they happen to be. We love our coffee in the morning, or in my case, tea. We eat a ton of bread and we never seem to tire of bacon. Even though we have an endless number of food options, humans tend to reach for what they know. If you think about it, that's pretty restrictive, even if you're the one who's making the choices. What you need is a new way to cook and eat that's good and satisfying, and doesn't involve my mother's favorite go-to recipes which start with, "Take a pound of butter."

This one didn't necessarily come easily to me. I spent a lot of time figuring out what to cook and how to cook it. Those methods will be discussed in a later chapter, but I will say this: now that I have a plan, my life is so much easier because I no longer have to agonize over that question, "What's for dinner?" because I have a plan.

I want to help people to properly learn to nourish their bodies, which is the furthest thing from restriction. If you are still restricting calories and over-exercising to lose weight, you will continue the battle of the bulge. You will eventually get fatter after each diet you are on. In fact, you are actually destroying your metabolism! The exact opposite of what you want to happen is happening by dieting. You will learn more about this in the coming chapters. The average American buys four diet books a year. I am determined to teach people the right way to never diet again and have the healthy body of their dreams. Prepare to never count another calorie. Say goodbye to "hangry", the combination of hungry and angry. Say hello to VITALITY and STRENGTH!

Before we go on, really stop and think about your attitudes toward food. Do you eat to nourish your body, or is there more involved?

What are some reasons you eat?

POWER VERSE:

"If you are willing and obedient, you will eat the good things of the land." -Isaiah 1:19 NIV

Chapter 12
I Don't Have Enough Self Control

If you can't get control of yourself, who should? If you are a parent, your kids are watching. More is caught than is taught.

I relate easily to this one. If you put a chocolate chip cookie in front of me I'm probably going to eat it. I've learned that the key here, again, is planning. It sounds simple. If you can't resist it, don't buy it. But that's not enough. What's needed is a plan and an attractive alternative that you can reach for when the urge for something gooey and delicious overtakes you. If you do that, chances are you'll learn to satisfy that urge without eating an entire tub of ice cream. Some people have other tricks that they use to stay on track. I have a friend who doesn't buy junk food to keep on hand, but if she truly craves something that may not be a good choice she has to walk to the grocery store to get it. The round trip is three miles. That's usually enough time for her to reconsider, but if it's not and she just has to have that chocolate cake, she's at least kept her metabolism revved while she satisfies the urge. And she never buys more than she can eat in one sitting. It also helps if you can get the whole family on board. Because my husband knows that I comfort myself with food, he used to buy candy for me when he thought I was feeling down. He's learning to console me with hugs instead. He also can't resist a bargain, so after Halloween, Christmas, or Easter he tends to stock up on leftover holiday treats. I scolded him the last time he did it, pointing out that I only have so much self-control and that neither of us needs that kind of thing, and the next day they disappeared. As I was bringing out the Christmas decorations this year I pulled out a box and a whole grocery bag of expired Cadbury Crème Eggs fell out on the floor. He'd hidden them around the house so they weren't there to tempt me, and then forgot about them.

It also helps to eat when you're hungry rather than starving. Again the key word here is planning.

"I don't have self-control" may just be another excuse or limited belief you have created. Two things could be happening when you are telling yourself this. Either you have created this belief so you can keep eating the crap and feel justified, or your blood sugar is dropping so low from going too long without eating that inevitably you are always choosing wrong because you're choosing from a position of weakness, biologically speaking. When your blood sugar is stable, you honestly don't crave the crap. But if you are waiting five hours in between meals, your blood sugar drops and your body begins to burn your muscle. You are starving! You could have the strength of Hercules and you would still fail because when you have low blood sugar, willpower goes out the window. So at that point you either reach for a dead carbohydrate (sugar, chips, pop) or you overeat because your hormone leptin (which tells you you're full) is out of whack from dieting and stress. It's time to stabilize your blood sugar. Watch all the videos at www.pfcevery3.com to help you understand blood sugar stabilization better. Homeostasis=PFC Every 3!

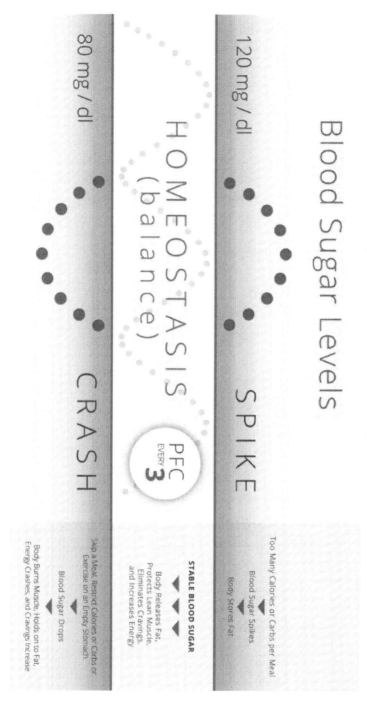

Photo by Venice Nutrition

Just remember, when you eat PFC (protein, fat, carb) every three hours, your blood sugar is stable and those crazy cravings will be gone! When the pain of staying the same becomes greater than the pain of change, you will change. That is why once someone has a heart attack and lives, they are more likely to work on getting healthy!

Hopefully you don't have to let your life get really bad before you make it good. Choose self-control. In coming chapters we will teach you to stabilize your blood sugar so you don't constantly have to be battling your cravings.

We'll help you to get control of yourself by eating PFC Every 3 and teach your children to do the same. When you take control of what you are putting into your mouth, you will raise up mentally stronger children who know how to nourish their bodies.

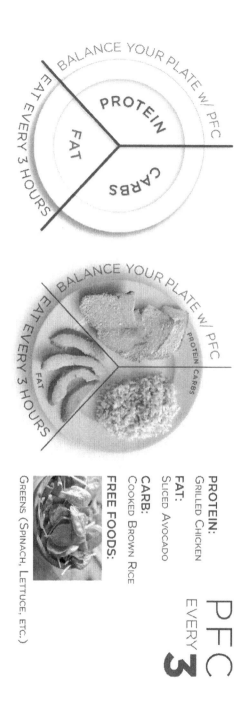

PROTEIN: GRILLED CHICKEN

FAT: SLICED AVOCADO

CARB: COOKED BROWN RICE

FREE FOODS: GREENS (SPINACH, LETTUCE, ETC.)

PFC
EVERY
3

Photo by Venice Nutrition

How many times are you eating per day?

_____

_____

What are your go-to foods?

_____

_____

List an example of a protein, fat and carb. If you're not sure, you're about to learn! This will be an easier exercise after you check out www.pfcevery3.com.

1. **Protein**_____
2. **Fat**_____
3. **Carb (living carb)**_____

POWER VERSE:

"For God has not given us a spirit of fear, but of power and of love and of a sound mind."-2 Timothy 1:7 NKJV

Chapter 13
Healthy Foods are Too Expensive

How much is your health worth? What's the cost of being unhealthy? Eating healthy can improve your quality of life and ultimately save you unnecessary costs related to being unhealthy later in life.

When I tried this one out on Renita she told me I was kidding myself, and then explained why this excuse doesn't fly. It's true that high quality, organic and fresh foods are more expensive than a box of macaroni and cheese or ramen noodles. But let's be honest with ourselves. Look at the receipt from your last trip to the grocery store. Go ahead, look. What did it include? Did you buy crackers, chips, soda, ice cream, cookies, candy, pre-packaged meals, and food from the delicatessen? Eliminate those foods and you'll find you have a whole lot more to spend on healthier options. Does this mean you won't enjoy your food in the future? Not at all. I've learned that it just means you need to prepare before you go to the grocery store and spend some time getting ready for the week ahead. We're going to show you how to do it.

Poor health is costing our country trillions every year. Obesity and overweight are directly linked to nearly 80% of our health problems. The co-pay on open heart surgery is $15,000. Cancer

costs some families tens of thousands out of pocket. Being healthy is cheap when compared to the cost of disease, not to mention the mental, emotional, and spiritual turmoil it causes families.

Why is junk food so cheap? Why can we buy 10 boxes of macaroni and cheese for a dollar. What is in it that it can be produced that cheaply? You pay for what you get.

Honestly, I believe people don't realize that the food we are consuming can either heal cell function *or* destroy our cells. The healthier the food we eat, the better our cell renewal and healing will be. It is called epigenetics (above genes)!

All the food we eat, supplements we take, water we drink, how much we move (or don't move) our bodies and the thoughts we think are all linked to preventing or causing disease. In fact, studies now show that as much as 80% of our health is influenced by epigenetics, factors outside of our basic DNA makeup that can change the way our cells function. The things we invest in to keep ourselves or our families well definitely matter. Think about that the next time you are buying 10 boxes of macaroni for a dollar. Not the best investment for your family's health.

Go to your cupboard right now and find 10 things your family would be better off without.

Get rid of it!

List the five foods you need to stop buying and start replacing with healthier options:

1._____

2._____

3._____

4._____

5._____

Here is a list to help you when you're grocery shopping:

1. Try to purchase 95% of your groceries in the outer parameters of the store. Don't go into the middle aisles as they are like a black hole and will suck you in!
2. Avoid ALL food with artificial colors. Blue, Red, Yellow which are mostly found in fruit snacks, soda, and most processed food.
3. Opt for low sodium alternatives, as you should have approximately 250 mg of sodium per meal.
4. Avoid hydrogenated or trans-fat. (This is the fat that is solid at room temperature found in MANY processed foods.)
5. When buying bread, always look for "whole" as the first ingredient. Always buy organic. I look for Three Bakers Bread, which is gluten free.
6. Avoid processed foods with "wheat gluten" and high-fructose corn syrup in them (bread, cereal, snack foods).
7. COLOR, COLOR, COLOR- ROYGBIV. Buy and eat all the colors of the rainbow in fresh fruits and vegetables!
8. Try to avoid nitrates and nitrites (in processed meats) which are linked to causing cancer.
9. Avoid aspartame, Splenda and sucralose. Substitute Stevia, raw honey, or coconut palm sugar.

10. Fresh (best), frozen (next best, especially if flash frozen with no added sugars or salts), canned (in moderation).
11. Raw nuts are your best choice.
12. When planning a meal make sure 51% of your plate is raw and living food, not tan, brown, or white.
13. PFC (protein, fat, carb) every three hours! To check out the program go to www.pfcevery3.com.
14. Spring water is best! (Drink at least 1/2 your body weight in ounces.)
15. Get to know the whole foods or organic foods department manager! Build a relationship, offer them information about why you choose certain brands and nicely suggest or request new options!
16. Always remember the ingredients are listed from the highest amount (first ingredient) to lowest amount (last ingredient).
17. The fewer the ingredients, the better!
18. Understanding Percent Daily Values on the label - 5% is considered low while 20% is high.
    a. The items you want to be low are trans fat and sodium
    b. The items you want to be high are dietary fiber and protein
19. Always buy products with low sugar- fewer than 12 g/serving (you only want approximately 35-45 g of sugar in an entire day).
20. Sugar should never comprise more than 1/3 of your total carbohydrates.
21. When comparing brands, or choosing food, buy one with the most fiber per serving.
22. Start thinking of your carbohydrates as brightly-colored fruits and vegetables.
23. Say NO to soda.

24. Buy organic when possible. How do you know if a product is organic? When reading a label, look for the PLU code. If the code begins with 9 it is organic produce. GMOs have a five digit code beginning with an 8. Conventional produce has a four digit code.
25. Shop for groceries when you are not hungry.

POWER VERSE:

"The angel went to her and said, "Greetings, you who are highly favored! The Lord is with you."-Luke 1:28 NIV

Chapter 14
I Can't Cook

The truth is, cooking is simple. Shifting your mindset to a "can do" attitude is imperative for you to begin to adequately plan.

I have been truly spoiled here. For most of my children's lives I didn't have to cook because my mother did the job for me. I worked until 7:00 most nights and when I got home, dinner was on the table. She started doing this after her husband died, both as a way to help out and because she also ate better when she had someone to cook for. It's only recently, as my children have grown and gone, that I've had to face the kitchen, and I've come to this conclusion: if you can read, you can cook, because all that's required is a recipe book and some basic tools. If you don't like it, you, like me, will have to adjust your attitude. Consider it an investment in yourself and in your family's health. It's not hard. If I can do it, you can do it.

When you say I can't cook or I don't like to cook, consider that at one time, you couldn't walk either. You couldn't add numbers. You couldn't tie your shoe. You couldn't drive a car. You get my point. Imagine if you hadn't taken the time to learn those skills. There are numerous tools out there to help you have success in the kitchen. Are you willing to take the time to

learn and apply them? If not, you will never truly experience abundant health.

Start with just a few healthy meals. Choose a protein, choose a fat, and choose a carbohydrate.

Seasoning is simple too. I love Mrs. Dash as it is low in sodium. I love onions and garlic, Himalayan sea salt, turmeric, pepper, and so many herbs and spices to dress up my meals.

A great resource to help you with meal ideas, recipes, and food prep is www.allstrongmoms.com.

Another place to check out is the All Strong Moms Facebook page. Go "like" it now!

What three healthy meals would you like to learn to cook?

1._____

2._____

3._____

Commit to buying a healthy recipe book, or easier yet, Google your recipe, and add the word "healthy."

Example: Google "healthy spaghetti." You will be amazed at what's available for you on the World Wide Web to help you get healthy.

POWER VERSE:

"Commit thy way unto the Lord; trust also in Him, and He shall bring it to pass." -Psalm 37:5 KJV

Chapter 15
I Don't Want to Cook Just for Myself

Cooking for one can be a lot of fun and can save you lots of money. If it's not fun at first, stick with it. The money you save can be used for... you guessed it...fun!

Try preparing a few days' or even the week's food all at once and be done with it, at least for a while. Or take a cue from my mother and help out a family in need with the extra that you prepare. If you actually sit down and think about what it costs to feed even one person with takeout or restaurant food every night, I think you'd be appalled. I know one person who challenged himself to cook at home by putting the money he saved every week into a vacation fund. When the year was over he went to Bali, something he'd always wanted to do. He became a gourmet cook in the process, too.

Also, consider what's actually *in* that restaurant food. You'll not only shave dollars off your food bill, you'll add years to your life.

I love the idea of cooking for others. In fact, cook *with* others! Have a Sunday meal prep day where you prepare extra food to freeze for yourself. If you are doing it with a few friends, it will

be fun! You can celebrate your day of food prepping with a meal for all of you. If you have extras, take it to a family of your choice. A new mom or a sick grandmother would appreciate a great meal! Take turns prepping food at each other's houses. Developing these healthy habits now will last a lifetime.

Who do you know who wants to start a healthy lifestyle and could start Sunday food prepping with me?

1._____

2._____

3._____

Who could you take a healthy meal to this week?

1._____

2._____

POWER VERSE:

"Share your food with the hungry, and give shelter to the homeless. Give clothes to those who need them, and do not hide from relatives who need your help." -Isaiah 58:7 NLT

Chapter 16
My Family Won't Eat It

Here's what I tell my boys all the time: "God gave me you to take the best possible care of you. He gave me you to nourish you, to love you, and to protect you. Eating healthy food is doing all those things. Thank God we *get* to be healthy!"

Try it! Most kids won't argue with what God says!

There's a magnet on my refrigerator that says, "What's for supper? Why, a big, heaping helping of EAT IT OR STARVE!" I bought that because I could relate. I think God gave me the world's pickiest eaters. In Central America, for instance, an awful lot of people subsist on rice, beans and tortillas and they're happy to get it. They don't worry that they've had the same thing to eat twice this week, or that chicken isn't their favorite. But here, our endless variety and the vast quantities of food with which we are blessed have given rise to extreme food preferences. Research says your best plan of attack is to start children out on healthy eating from the womb, but if that train has already left the station for you, I can only suggest leading by example and learning how to cook foods that are attractive and truly taste good. Child nutrition experts insist that a child must be exposed to a new food 16 times before he or she stops viewing it with suspicion and actually reaches for it, so start them early if you can. And if you can't, take heart from the research that shows our taste buds become more sophisticated as we age.

"My family won't eat it" is an excuse you use to not prepare healthy food. Far too many moms are hijacked by their children's opinions of food. Most kids would prefer to live on sugar and colorful things, like Fruity Pebbles. Tell yourself, "Not on my watch." Our kids don't buy the groceries, we do. Studies show kids need to be exposed 11 to 18 times before they try it, or better yet, like it. Keep insisting they try just a bite.

Here is some simple advice: quit buying unhealthy food! If you make the food taste great, make the preparation fun, and include them in the process of change, they will eat healthy, nourishing food.

My husband Scott and I include our three boys in our cooking so they can live healthy, active lives! They are all learning early and were able to cook their own eggs by the time they were six years old. We knew we were on to something when our oldest son Beau, now 16, asked for an omelet pan for his sixth birthday! It was simply a choice we made to include our boys in the process. Our children have to learn to eat right because they have to do it for the rest of their lives. We will teach and train them while they're young to nourish themselves, and hopefully they will be proactive with their health as they get older.

As a mom, it is much easier to train them when they are five than when they are 50. If they're hungry, they will eventually eat what they're given. When I have made food changes in my family, it hasn't always been easy. There were even tears and name calling a few times. I knew it would be challenging, but I also knew it would be worth it.

But as you can see with Monica, even a beautiful, busy woman in her 50s can create change in the home. It can be done at any age. You must make a decision that you are worth it, and so is your family!

Encourage your family to have fun making a healthy meal with you this week. www.allstrongmoms.com will help.

Think of three healthy meals. Kids like choices.

1._____

2._____

3._____

POWER VERSE:

"Start children off in the way they should go, and even when they are old they will not turn from it." -Proverbs 22:6 NIV

Chapter 17
Exercise is Boring

Eighty percent of weight loss is nutrition and 20% is exercise. That 20% is crucial as you get older! A complaint I hear often is "Exercise is boring!" If that is the case, you are not really exercising. Everything about exercise is stimulating your body, mind, and spirit. If it is boring, you are more than likely doing it improperly. I am always invigorated and refreshed after a healthy workout.

It's true what they say – you don't appreciate something until you no longer have it. This is certainly the case with exercise. If you're fortunate and you work at it, you can live a healthy and active life long into your 80s and 90s, but most of us have to work at it. How you live and what you're able to do as you age will be determined largely by what you do now to build a healthy foundation. A walk around the golf course may not sound so appealing until you're truly unable to lift yourself out of a chair to do it. Sitting in front of the TV day in and day out because you really can't do anything else is the definition of boring. So get up and go walking, biking, bowling, golfing, snow shoeing, skiing, running, boating, gardening – do yoga, play tennis, throw a ball – whatever it takes to get you up and moving. Life is fun when you feel good!

If you're bored with workouts and you're looking for great results with some major variety and fun, a great place to start is www.allstrongmoms.com! If you're getting up in age or haven't worked out in years there is a great option at that website called ALL STRONG GRANDMOMS! Our healthy bodies are built in the kitchen with great nutrition, but your strength will increase as you undertake the compounding effect of doing a little more with every workout. Ideally, try to strength train two to three times a week to improve your muscular strength and endurance. Eventually, the workout that is kicking your butt will be your warm-up.

Every time you work out, you create micro trauma to your muscle tissue and your muscles rebuild themselves stronger and better than they were before. Proper nutrition will work to fuel your workouts and enhance the results you are looking for. When you are eating correctly, your body recovers faster and quickly becomes stronger. When you aren't eating correctly, it seems as if it takes forever to recover from a workout. With working out, you are eating for performance.

When you strengthen your body, you enjoy amazing mental and emotional breakthroughs as well. Remember, motion releases emotion. In fact, the mental and emotional benefits of exercise may even surpass the physical!

POWER VERSE:

"... But the people who know their God shall stand firm and take action." -Daniel 11:32 ESV

Chapter 18
I'm Too out of Shape

One of the biggest obstacles when beginning exercise is the F.A.T. (Far Away from Truth) excuse that you are too out of shape to start.

In 1986, about six weeks after I gave birth to my daughter, Meghanne, my assignment editor at KMVT-TV told me he wanted me to take part in a class on rappelling in the Sawtooth Mountains. If you've seen Idaho's Sawtooths, you know that they're high up there, and I hate heights. I can't even look over the edge of tall buildings because of what that does to my stomach: that flip-flop sensation that leads to hyperventilation. I hate carnival rides. I want my hotel rooms to be on the ground floor. My idea of a nightmare is a roller coaster. But, I didn't want my boss to think I wasn't willing to go the extra mile, so I kept my misgivings to myself and with Cliff as my photographer, I started out for bear country. I figured it was a beginner class, so how bad could it be?

Let me tell you how bad. First was the six-mile hike to get to the rock face that we were going to climb. The instructor was the winner of the Iron Man competition and he wasn't inclined to baby anybody, including Cliff, who had to make the trek carrying 50 pounds of camera gear. We definitely brought up the rear.

When we got to our destination the instructor told us, boot camp style, to do exactly what he said so we wouldn't get hurt. Then he pointed out the chosen rock face. It was sheer, shiny granite and to me, looked nearly vertical. Our first order of business was to remove our shoes and socks. As we did, he explained that even though the rock felt smooth, it was actually rough in spots and if we found the rough patches and stood straight up, gravity would keep us on the mountain. As soon as we gave in to fear, though, and tried to hug the rock, we'd fall. I was expecting to wear a rope, but that was for later. Our baby steps would be taken barefoot and (here came the surprise) blindfolded. That way, he reasoned, we wouldn't give in to the temptation to look down and slide. We would be doing the work by sheer feel.

Four hours later we stopped for lunch, our feet bleeding and our thighs trembling with exhaustion. However, we were all able to stand upright on that rock without sliding. After lunch (and I'll admit, a quick snooze), we donned the ropes and began the real climb. This time we took turns being the climber and the belayer, the person holding the rope. I wanted to take comfort from the fact that the rope was around me, except that I knew the person holding the other end was just as inexperienced as I was. But then I looked up and saw Cliff and his camera above me. Somehow, he had made the climb while carrying the camera gear so I figured I could do it carrying just my water bottle. And as an added bonus, I got to keep my shoes on. Later I found out Cliff had gone around by a different, less steep route, but I didn't know it at the time.

The entire time I was climbing that rock I was telling myself that as soon as I got back down on the ground, if I ever did, I was going to get a job as a Walmart greeter; anything where I got to keep my feet firmly planted. Once at the top, though, the instructor, who was beside me the entire time, told me to turn around and look. And there I was, on top of the world. I had done a hard physical thing and when it was over I felt proud of myself in a way you can't feel unless you have faced down your fear. So, remembering that experience, I thought to myself, what's a little running?

Now, this was 20 years later and I was about to scale an entirely different mountain. I was about to run a 5K. I was older, heavier, and severely out of shape. But I knew I had to start. If I didn't I would continue down the path of obesity and sickness.

You are never too old or too out of shape to start! I work with people in their 80s and 90s who are just "starting" their exercise program. I also work with the morbidly obese and I can confidently say you are never too far gone to start an exercise program. Many times we start by just doing things seated. Gradually you are stronger and healthier and will surprise yourself with your new strength and range of motion. Bottom line...JUST DO IT!

Many women tell me they are too out of shape to go to my exercise class, or they're going to get into better shape before they come to the class. Just think for one minute how crazy that sounds. Isn't that the purpose of exercise, to get you into shape? When you exercise it creates positive stress in order to strengthen your cardiovascular and muscular systems, as well as bone density. The secret to seeing results is doing something persistently and consistently. Many people exercise for one month and expect to have an entire body makeover after raising hell with their bodies for 30 years. I guarantee if you exercise consistently for three months, your body and health will improve drastically. That is exactly why I created www.millionstepchallenge.com. It gives you a daily goal of 11,111 steps per day for 90 days. There are also amazing weekly workouts with the PLUS version!

I have told Monica and so many other women over the years, you are more than a number on a scale. All that number does is give us a direction of where we need to go and what we need to do. On your health journey, it is best to focus on those positive daily choices you are making that will eventually become habits. The number on the scale will be exactly where you want it to be when you have a mind and heart shift. Your weight is influenced by your beliefs and is a by-product of your nutrition and fitness decisions. You are beautiful, healthy, strong and courageous. God says so. Start living like it with the appropriate actions.

The secret is getting your actions aligned with what God believes about you. You may have been lying to yourself for years or abusing yourself verbally. Instead, choose to love yourself. You are wonderfully made. You are a conqueror! You can experience abundant health!

Here's an exercise that will help you get started by changing your excuses to positive reasons. Your positive reasons will become your new beliefs!

Make two columns. On one side write your limiting beliefs or excuses. For example: "I don't have time to exercise." On the other side, write your new belief. In this case, "I choose to make time to exercise because I love getting healthy." When you have your two lists, go back and circle the New Belief column with a red pen and make a big X through those limiting beliefs and excuses that are no longer serving your best interests.

Limiting Belief	New Belief
I don't have time.	I choose to make time!
I hate exercise.	I love getting healthy!

POWER VERSE:

"Finally brothers and sisters, whatever is true, whatever is noble, whatever is right, whatever is pure, whatever is lovely, whatever is admirable- if anything is excellent or praiseworthy- think about such things." -Philippians 4:8 NIV

Chapter 19
I Focus on My Weight, Not on My Health

Have you noticed the "health food" section in the grocery store? Most have them now. What does that make the rest of the food in the store? Do you get it?

The first thing Renita did was talk about my health. She said health was a combination of many things: weight, measurements, blood pressure, pH, bone density, body fat and so much more. On day one she asked me (no, she forced me) to step on the scale. She measured me, checked my pH levels, recorded how much water I had in my body and got a reading on my bone density. We talked about nutrition for a long time and she suggested that I should not start out running right away. She told me I'd have better success if I first lost some of the excess weight I was carrying. To illustrate, she dressed me in a weighted vest and had me walk around her neighborhood with her. Carrying that extra 10 pounds had me puffing like a steam engine in no time. It was much easier to do the walking without that vest, and I could immediately see her point, that running would also be easier if I was lighter. Health is about nourishing my body, not abusing it. The eating program we followed was PFC Every 3.

The plan is not a diet. Rather, it's a new way of eating that actually takes us back to infancy. A newborn baby demands to be fed every two or three hours and Lord help you if you ignore their cries. Ask me how I know. My oldest was born at a time when schedules were still a thing when it came to parenting a newborn. All of the experts of the day told me that if I didn't put her on a schedule I'd be spoiling her. So, I watched the clock, waiting for the three-hour mark while she screamed, and screamed, and screamed. Ten years elapsed between my first and my last, and by the time Hannah came along I didn't worry about time at all. When she cried, I fed her, and she was a much happier baby. We can all learn a lesson from this. Nature still intends us to eat that way.

Now consider breast milk. It contains the perfect balances of protein, fat and carbohydrates. As we grow out of infancy, the way we get that mix and the foods we eat change, but the basic biology remains the same. We need protein, fat and carbs every three hours in order to keep our metabolism firing. The PFC Every 3 Zen Program developed by Mark Macdonald (author of *Body Confidence* and *Why Kids Make You Fat*) is based on that principle, and it's the eating plan that Renita taught me. She is a certified nutrition coach.

Renita and I started with a detox phase which I thought I'd done before. But really, what I'd done before was starve myself. A lot of diets talk about detox, but I have learned there is a right way and a wrong way to go about it. Detox is not about going hungry. Rather, it's about clearing your body of bloat by eliminating toxins, which in my case came initially from a whole lot of NutraSweet and a diet that for years was based mainly on grains and sugar. With the PFC Every 3 program, detox had me eating "clean" foods, along with supplements and drinking a lot of water. The idea was, as Renita put it, to drain the dirty bathwater before we got started. The detox phase was quickly gratifying because I took off seven pounds right away. Over the course of the next few weeks I lost a little more, and before we started training, the first 10 pounds were gone. Honestly, the only exercise I did during detox was walking and breathing (as breathing helps to eliminate toxins along with the sweating).

Detox was over and the training for the 5K was about to begin. Remembering that walk around the block with the ten pound weighted vest, I thought I would be pretty fleet-footed. Just to be sure though, I snuck over to the indoor track without Renita. I wanted to be alone for that first run.

On the track I chose, one lap is a ninth of a mile. That means I had to run it nine times to equal mile. I made it halfway around once before my chest burned and my heart started to pound. I had to walk the rest of the way. Armed with my asthma rescue inhaler I went back the next night, and the next, until I could at least make it all the way around one time at a shuffling jog. It was at about this point that my daily workouts with Renita started. She fit me with a heart monitor so I could tell how hard I was working, how many calories I was burning and how much progress I was making. It was a great motivator because I could actually see improvement from day to day. By the end of the first month I was running a half mile. By the second, it was a mile, and by the third it was two miles. At the same time, we were focusing on strength training. The progress there seemed slower to me, mainly because I couldn't see immediate results. My muscles were getting stronger, but they were buried in fat so I couldn't see them. Renita did, though, and her encouragement along with daily workouts, nutrition tracking, good food and falling dress sizes kept me going until I really could see a big difference in the mirror.

I was not in tip-top condition, but I was no longer "too out of shape to even start." I was no longer "toxic." I was definitely on the road to better health!

I have an awesome friend and client, Leota. She is 80 and has completely changed her life, losing 100 pounds! She even carries her own salad dressing with her to the restaurant. She could

have said, "I am too old. I don't know what to do. I use a walker to get around. I am 100 pounds overweight." Instead, she said, "I am sick of being overweight and sick! I am sick of feeling lethargic and old!" When she took charge of what she was eating, her doctor took her off her blood pressure and diabetes medications within three weeks of implementing the PFC Every 3 plan!

Remember this: what you currently eat is what you will crave. So if you are eating sugar, fast food, or soda, those are what you'll want. Don't trust only your "feelings" or "cravings" when it comes to proper nourishment while you are getting your health on track. Feelings are fickle and cravings are usually nutritional deficiencies or low blood sugar. Eventually, what we eat will positively affect our emotions. The cravings will diminish once we stabilize our blood sugar with PFC Every 3! To begin the change, especially if addicted to processed foods, it is important to follow a plan. When you begin eating healthy foods, you will begin craving those healthy, living, colorful foods. Eat alive, feel alive! Say that out loud a few times: "I choose to eat alive so I feel alive!"

What foods do you crave? Write them down and consider their nutritional value.

_____

_____

Besides your weight, what areas of your health would you like to improve?

_____

_____

POWER VERSE:

"But the Lord is with me like a mighty warrior."-Jeremiah 20:11

Chapter 20
No More Bingo Arms

You have seen them -- people at the bingo parlor waving their arms in the air, while their loose underarms seem to be chasing their hands.

"Nobody likes to look at a fat news anchor." That was what came out of Monica's mouth when she began. "I am not getting any younger. I am good at what I do, but let's face it, being healthy is in. Sleeveless tops with toned arms are what America wants. I want to be healthy with toned arms! Even more important is training for the 5K that I told our entire viewing audience I was going to do."

Even though Monica was overweight and felt that her best health and body were behind her, I was about to turn her life upside down. I knew from her confidence and competitive spirit that this goal was the awakening of her health and her best body ever!

I have realized from working with thousands of women and men that to get our physical body in shape, we must shift our mind and to get in alignment with the Holy Spirit. That is true wholeness. That is health. Monica just wanted to be able to run the 5K without dying. Instead, she was embarking on an empowering adventure that will last the rest of her life!

Ironically, Monica and I were on the cover of the *INSPIRE* magazine nearly 14 years ago as the Women of Inspiration for the year, she in media and me in fitness. Here we were again, our paths crossing. I always believe the second time you meet someone, it is for the real God-intended reason. The first go around was the warm up. I was honored that Monica chose me to help her get healthy and rock that 5k!

You don't know where you are going unless you figure out where you are. So after a brief health question and answer session, we began with weighing and measuring. The beauty is that even though that first time is nearly unbearable for women, it is the worst it will ever get when they come to me. From that day forward they see progress, improvement, strength, and yes improved numbers on the scale and tape measure. There are tears, shrieks, and excuses falling like raindrops as they peel off the layers of clothes and jewelry and step on the scale to be weighed. That wedding ring has to weigh at least a half a pound.

One thing you should know right from the start is you will never out-work a bad diet. As stated earlier, nutrition is nearly 80% of weight loss and overall health. Fitness is only about 20% of losing weight! It was clear to me that Monica was swollen. She was bloated, toxic, and tired from carrying around all that extra weight. I told her, "First things first, we have got to detox! This will cleanse your colon, liver, and kidneys." The healthy questionnaire pointed out all the things holding her back. She told me that her knee hurt, especially when she was playing tennis, so she had quit playing. Knowing that training for a 5K would involve some running, I knew we had to strip off about 25 pounds to lighten the impact not only on her knee, but on her entire body, including her mind.

As a Certified Venice Nutrition Coach, I follow an amazing program that teaches people to detox, ignite, and thrive. It is called Zen Project 8, created by my friend and mentor, Mark

Macdonald. He is the *New York Times* best-selling author of *Why Kids Make you Fat and How to Get Your Body Back.* By stabilizing your blood sugar, you literally turn on your metabolism. Our state, North Dakota, has lost over 63,000 pounds of fat with this plan! You can check it out by going to my website www.pfcevery3.com.

   Detox consists of getting rid of the bloat by flushing the toxins from the body with amazing whole food nutrition, lots of water, and utilizing some natural herbs to cleanse the colon, liver, and kidneys. Detox really is like draining the dirty bath water before climbing into the tub. It was imperative that we start there with Monica, as she had just quit drinking Diet Coke. She typically had six to 10 cans per day and drank absolutely NO water. That was another part of the detox: cleansing and flushing her body with plenty of spring water. In fact, I told her she would need to drink half her body weight in ounces of water daily. A week later she showed me the trunk of her car. It had *cases* of bottled spring water in it. The best part – it was spring in North Dakota so her car had lots of natural refrigeration. I love a teachable spirit!

   Another great component needed to improve Monica's nutrition was to actually eat. She had been living on caffeine from the Diet Coke and eating only two meals a day. By doing this, she actually slowed her metabolic rate. Eating only a few times a day or skipping meals doesn't make you thinner, it makes you fatter. I told her, "If you skip a meal, it is like you are working on getting fatter because it is slowing down your metabolic rate." It's not surprising that she was eating this way because that is how the diet industry has taught us to eat – calories in vs. calories out. Eat less, move more. Eat only 1,200 calories a day or worse yet, don't eat at all. Just drink concoctions. Stop eating at 5 pm. Eliminate all carbs. Eat only cabbage soup. Eat only grapefruit. Eat only meat. Recognize any of these?

   The truth is the diet industry is designed to fail you. It's a big, fat lie! Its leaders want you to lose weight quickly by doing crazy things and, worse yet, feeling crazy while you are doing them. The key to successful weight loss isn't calories. The key is stabilizing your blood sugar to ignite your metabolism. This will literally turn your body into a fat burning machine. We have starved ourselves fat as a nation and it's time to wake up and eat. Literally, wake up and eat! I knew at the age of 55 Monica had caused her metabolism to stagnate and she was staying afloat with her caffeine buzz. After she had hung up the Diet Coke, the real work began. The goal was to get her natural metabolism back. I knew she would be literally forcing herself to eat during detox and from the sound of it, she would start pooping again.

Her digestive system was a mess, with chronic constipation followed by bouts of diarrhea. She had a distended belly and there was no hiding it. It was time to deflate the balloon. Is caffeine helping you get through your day? Are you pooping at least two times a day? Are you ready to feel amazing from your nutrition and to poop like a goose so your belly is never distended?

POWER VERSE:

"But because of his great love for us, God who is rich in mercy, made us alive with Christ even when we were dead in our transgressions- it is by grace you have been saved." -Ephesians 2:4-5 NIV

Chapter 21
PFC Every 3 Like a Baby

In America, we have a big problem. Ours is the land of the fad diet and the mindset that we can achieve spot reduction with "this simple exercise." Perhaps you've heard that you can "spray your fat away, freeze your fat away, and suck your fat away." In plain English, we have dieted ourselves fat and spot-reduced ourselves silly. It comes down to this: 80 percent of our health, weight loss, and vitality is generated by the nutrients we put into our mouths. If we are putting the wrong nutrients in, we are going to have a tough time reaching our goals.

Anyone can lose weight for a little while. Think of people you know who have dieted themselves thinner, but when you see that person three months later they're fatter than ever! This happens because you actually increase your set-point weight every time you diet. Not to mention that it is hugely stressful on our arterial walls and can lead to heart disease. The truth about nutrition is that you need the following for your cells to function properly: macronutrients, micronutrients, phytonutrients, essential fats, and water. If you are missing any of these your weight loss is temporary, not to mention you don't feel alive and well. That is why so many diets fail. They eliminate one or more of these and as a result, our bodies are nutrient deficient, which leads to crazy cravings. In addition, every deficiency must eventually be replenished or disease will occur. Go to www.pfcevery3.com to have a clear understanding of the nutrients our bodies need to have amazing health!

So what is "PFC Every 3 like a baby?" PFC stands for protein, fat and carbohydrates. "Every 3 like a baby" refers to getting back to the first and possibly last time we perfectly nourished our bodies. Eating the right portion sizes of protein, healthy fat, and colorful living carbohydrates every three hours is how your body will get back on track for good!

Let's start with a simple science lesson.

Nutrients are the substances we need for growth and they are fuels that drive our bodily functions.

Macronutrients are the building blocks that provide calories or energy. Since "macro" means large, macronutrients are the nutrients we need in large amounts. There are three macronutrients:

- Protein
- Fat
- Carbohydrates

Why Do We Need Protein?

- Growth (especially for children, teens, and pregnant women)
- Tissue repair
- Immune function
- Making essential hormones and enzymes
- Energy when carbohydrates are not available
- Preserving lean muscle mass and building lean muscle mass, which is super important as you age

Protein is found in:

- Meats
- Poultry
- Fish
- Eggs
- Cheese
- Milk
- Nuts
- Legumes
- And in smaller quantities in vegetables

When we eat these types of foods, our body breaks down the protein that they contain into amino acids, which are the building blocks of proteins. Some amino acids are essential, which means that we need to get them from our diet. Others are nonessential, which means that our body can make them on its own. Protein that comes from animal sources contains all of the essential amino acids that we need and are called "complete proteins." Plant sources of protein, on the other hand, do not contain all of the essential amino acids and are called "incomplete proteins."

With the PFC Every 3 program, complete proteins are what we refer to as "P." Nuts, beans, and most vegetables will *not* count as our protein source as they lack some essential amino acids.

1/3 of your plate should be complete proteins.

For your complete protein sources eat :

- Organic grass fed beef
- Bison
- Chicken
- Fish

- Turkey
- Eggs
- Organic cheese
- Organic milk (raw is best)
- Kefir

These complete proteins help build and maintain that lean muscle as you age!

Do We Need Fat?

Fat is essential for survival! Over the years, many Americans have gone fat free or low fat, and the crazy thing is, our country is fatter than ever. Clearly, this strategy and teaching is a complete failure. There are healthy fats and unhealthy fats. Healthy, nourishing fats are necessary for good health and will allow our bodies to release stored fat! If you are not eating enough nourishing fat, your weight loss will be stagnant. In addition, by going fat free or low fat, you will never permanently achieve your health and weight loss goals.

Fat is crucial for many reasons. One of the biggest is that it aids in weight loss by helping us feel satisfied. In addition, we feel full longer. Have you ever eaten something that's fat free, say a carb like licorice for example, and walked away still hungry? You could down the entire bag and it still wouldn't be enough to truly satisfy you. Nourishing fats will help you to lose that extra fat on your body and will also help you to feel full. Healthy fat makes up our cell walls so that we have better cellular communication which leads to a better metabolism! Fat also has the following benefits:

- Promotes normal growth and development
- Gives increased energy (fat is the most concentrated source of energy)

- Enables the absorption of certain vitamins (like vitamins A, D, E, K, and carotenoids)
- Provides cushioning for the organs
- Maintains cell membranes
- Provides taste, consistency, and stability to foods

You find nourishing fat in:

- Meat
- Poultry
- Fish
- Eggs
- Nuts
- Nut butters
- Milk products
- Organic butters
- Olive oil
- Coconut oil
- Avocado oil

There are three main types of fat:

- Saturated fat
- Unsaturated fat
- Trans fat (processed is the worst)

The main fat you need to avoid is trans fat, because our bodies cannot break it down appropriately. In addition, processed trans fats are directly linked to heart disease, cancer, obesity, weight gain, diabetes, and several other diseases. Other names for trans fats are hydrogenated fats or partially hydrogenated fats. Look at your labels and if you see either of these, get rid of it. You'll find it on countless foods, including snack crackers, bars, chips, nuts, cookies, fast food, and pretty much anything processed.

Just remember, all chemicals that your body cannot break down are being stored in your fat cells. Processed hydrogenated fats are linked to heart disease, because they create damage and plaque in the arterial walls. If your belly continues to expand, and your blood pressure and cholesterol continue to go up, it may be time for a detox!

1/3 of your plate should be healthy, nourishing fats.

Why Do We Need Carbohydrates?

Carbohydrates are a major energy source. Among other benefits, they make us feel happy. Without carbs, a person becomes crabby and lethargic. All carbohydrates are not created equal. Many are man-made, extremely processed, and our bodies simply do not recognize them or know how to digest them properly. High fructose corn syrup, processed grains and pastas, and candy are good examples of what I call "dead carbs," because they provide little nutritional benefit. They are typically devoid of most vitamins and minerals because of high heat and processing. Generally you will see words like, "enriched," because after heating has killed most of the nutrients, manufacturers try to add some nutritional value back in. Avoid these foods.

Living carbs, on the other hand, contain plenty of vitamins, minerals and enzymes.

With the PFC Every 3 program we consume mostly living carbs.

- Living carbohydrates are one of the body's main sources of fuel.
- Living carbohydrates are easily used by the body for energy.

- Living carbohydrates are needed for the central nervous system, the kidneys, the brain, and the muscles (including the heart) to function properly.
- Living carbohydrates can be stored in the muscles and liver and later used for energy.
- Living carbohydrates are important in intestinal health and waste elimination.

The best sources of living carbohydrates are found in:

- **Organic fruits**
- **Vegetables**
- **Beans**
- **Quinoa**
- **Brown rice**
- **Oats**
- **Sweet potatoes**
- **Sprouted grains**

Through my education and experience, I have found that people who consume LIVING carbs are setting themselves up for victory! Eat alive, feel alive!

Stay away from wheat gluten and processed grains. Gluten comes from the Latin word glue! It also means "any sticky substance." Is it any wonder that your belly continues to grow when you are eating breads and pastas? These foods are literally sticking to your colon wall and making you fatter and sicker, as well as constipated! If you don't believe me, give it up for two weeks and see how you feel. You will literally think more clearly!

Fiber refers to certain types of carbohydrates that our body cannot digest. These carbohydrates pass through the intestinal tract without breaking down and help move waste out of the body. Most vegetables and fruits are loaded with fiber. Diets low in fiber have been shown to cause problems such as constipation and hemorrhoids and increase the risk of certain types of cancer such as those of the colon. Diets high in fiber, however, have been shown to decrease your risk for heart disease and obesity, and help to lower your cholesterol.

1/3 of your plate should be living carbohydrates, which include foods high in fiber. Include a large salad with most meals. Dark, leafy greens are loaded with nutrients, plus dietary fiber. Leafy greens are considered a "free food," meaning you can eat as much as you like.

PFC Every 3 like a baby will set you free! If you can actually eat in that order P, F, C, your body will thank you! Check out www.pfcplate.com, a great tool that will help you with your weight loss and overall health process. It is super cool and will make learning to eat healthy super simple!

For more information on an exact grocery shopping list, meal plan, and how to lose approximately 20-42 lbs in 8 weeks, check out www.pfcevery3.com and its three phases of "Detox, Ignite, and Thrive." The best part about losing the weight with PFC Every 3 is you will know how to nourish your body and turn on your metabolism for life!

Finish this statement: PFC Every ___ like a _____ !

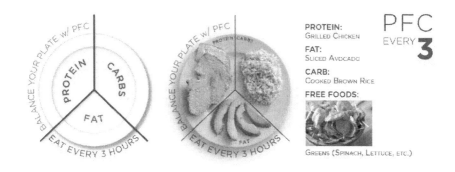

Photo by Venice Nutrition

POWER VERSE:

"Do you not know that your bodies are temples of the Holy Spirit, who is in you, who you have received from God?" -1 Corinthians 6:19 NIV

Chapter 22
The Key is in the Preparation

If you don't plan and prep your food, you are planning to fail.

To me, the three scariest words in the English language are "What's for dinner?" For years I managed to avoid the phrase by working at night. We went through eating phases. At first, when Cliff and I were newlyweds and he did most of the cooking we ate from boxes. A lot of Hamburger Helper passed through our systems. This may not sound like a health food, but compared to what I ate in college it was a definite step up. Then there was the frozen meal phase. We tended to like the single serving "diet" meals, although we could stretch a frozen lasagna for an entire week. I eventually got tired of this and we graduated to the Crock-Pot phase. We'd throw meat, potatoes or rice, and root vegetables in the pot in the morning and at night we'd eat stew. It didn't matter what the ingredients were, to me it always tasted like stew. When I got tired of that we were heading back in the direction of the boxed meals again and my mother finally stepped in. She thought what we were calling dinner was downright criminal. I couldn't have asked for a better deal, and it lasted for years. After my two oldest children moved away and the schedules for the rest of us became overly complicated, she stopped doing the cooking because she never knew who would be around. I was sad to see that go. Once again, the cooking chore was back on my lap.

So why did I hate the "What's for dinner" question? Because I never knew. I am not a good planner when it comes to the weekly menus. I tend not to think about it until I'm hungry. Of course that doesn't work for a busy family. We ended up eating a lot of spaghetti because it was fast. It didn't help that the three of us who remained in the household are all picky eaters.

When Renita agreed to train me, she didn't just hand me some weights or give me a workout routine to follow. She asked what I was eating, really listened, and then took me shopping. We avoided the middle of the store, staying instead on the perimeter of the supermarket where the whole foods and staples tend to be. She pointed out that the middle of the store is where the junk food and convenience foods are stocked. We prowled the whole foods and organic sections while she pointed out what she eats, why she likes it and why it works for a busy family. I noted that the prices were a bit higher. She, in turn, asked how much my health was worth. She wasn't letting me make any more excuses.

A short time after that she invited me over for an evening workout and as I did squats and leg lifts she asked me what I do to prepare for the week ahead in terms of food. I think I gave her a blank stare. That's when she said, "So how's that working for you?"

"Not so well," I readily admitted.

"You need to have a plan! You won't be successful otherwise," she insisted, and she brought me into her kitchen to show me what she meant. There, lined up on her counter, were dozens of foil packets with white fish, cut veggies, and spices. She had me make one so I'd get the idea cemented in my head, and then she insisted that I take three of the packets home for my family. I didn't have the heart to tell her that I never eat fish, nor does Hannah. Cliff ate all three! But the lesson made sense. If you have cut vegetables, hummus and healthy guacamole in your fridge, you're much less likely to reach for a bag of chips when you want a snack. If, on Sunday, you cook a dozen chicken breasts, wash and cut up vegetables, hard boil eggs and grill nitrate free turkey bacon, you're set for the week. Food that's mostly prepared means my family is much more likely to make a healthy lunch of turkey and veggie lettuce wraps during the next week. And when I come home from work tired, "hangry," and short on time, it's actually easier to toss together a stir fry of already cooked chicken and cut-up veggies than it is to go out again for fast food or to order and wait for a pizza. It's cheaper, too.

Since that first meal, Renita has fed me dozens of times. It's part of her mission because she knows how bad my old eating habits were. She's making sure I develop new ones. The food is always delicious and always different. She's an excellent and inventive cook and she doesn't mind sharing her secrets. Fresh, organic ingredients and spices are the keys to her success, and they can be the keys to yours as well.

Whatever You Do, Don't Skip Breakfast!

As for me, one of the big changes I've made has been to incorporate a healthy breakfast into my daily life and the lives of my family. We all used to skip breakfast. Now I make smoothies, or we eat hardboiled eggs with fruit. I also make egg "muffins," tossing cut up veggies, lean meat and eggs into muffin cups with a little cheese and bake them the night before. It's a quick-fix method she taught me. In the morning you just warm them up and presto, you are out the door! Greek yogurt is quick and doesn't require any preparation. Toss in a little fruit and some chia seeds and you're good to go.

I can remember telling people that I was never hungry in the mornings *unless* I ate breakfast. I assumed, as I'm sure many of you do, that by missing this meal I would be saving up calories for later. This classic mistake was probably responsible for more of my excess pounds than anything else. My body was actually trying to tell me something. Basic biology tells us we're supposed to eat regularly, and when I did, I felt hungry by mid-morning for a good reason. My metabolism was revved up. When I wasn't hungry, the opposite was happening: my metabolism was limping along. No wonder my dieting efforts were failing! I was starving my body and it was in self-preservation mode, just like a bear in hibernation. It was a huge relief when food stopped being the enemy. This mama bear was out of the cave.

Breakfast means break the fast. It literally kick starts your metabolism for the day. In fact, if you eat a PFC (protein, fat, carb) for breakfast, it is like putting a log in the fireplace. Your metabolism is hot, your body is burning fat, and your mind is clear. Several studies show that consuming protein first thing in the morning increases the speed of your metabolism!

An example of the perfect PFC: two scrambled eggs with some fresh cilantro, onions, tomatoes, and a little Mrs. Dash along with a fist full of berries!

I can identify how healthy and efficient your metabolism is by whether or not you are hungry first thing upon waking. Someone with a sluggish metabolism can go until noon without being hungry. It is time to turn on your metabolism by breaking that fast from the night of sleeping! When Monica eventually (after three months) showed up and told me she was waking at 5 a.m. STARVING, we did a happy dance! Her metabolism had fired back up. Three months of doing the right thing and that baby reignited

Do you eat breakfast?

Why or why not?

What do you eat for breakfast?

Is this a P, F, C?

POWER VERSE:

"'I have the right to do anything,' you say- but not everything is beneficial." -1 Corinthians 6:12 NIV

Chapter 23
Get off the Couch

I believe we can learn to love exercise. Not just the activity, but the byproducts of it: a clearer mind, a better attitude, more muscle tone as we age, and stronger bones. I know many individuals who are waiting for that perfect moment to begin an exercise program. Don't wait, start today!

Every weekend at my church the pastor invites the children to come forward with their gifts while the ushers pass the offering baskets. I can't help but smile watching the tiny bodies flying down the central aisle at a run, most of them grinning, looking proud to be handling this chore on their own. It struck me that children often run from place to place. When Dad comes in the door at night they launch themselves at him. They chase each other from room to room. On the playground they run from swing to slide. Just watching all of that energy can feel exhausting. It's almost as if once they acquire the skill, they want to put as many miles on as they can, as quickly as possible.

Early in my fitness journey, Renita and I started visiting playgrounds. My first job was to move hand-over-hand across the monkey bars. Moments before I tried it, a little boy shot past me and scurried across without giving it a second thought. I, on the other hand, could not swing my weight from one bar to the next.

Not even one time. I could barely hang from the bar. It's clear from watching children play that our bodies are designed to take us easily from one task to another, but by the time most of us have reached middle age our modern conveniences and sedentary jobs have done a number on us to the point where too often we can no longer comfortably carry our own weight.

The thing I learned over my months of training for my 5k and beyond is that you can redevelop those abilities. Even if you can't get back to the level where you can swing yourself across the monkey bars with the ease of a child, you are never too old to improve your physical fitness. I have also discovered that the world is full of people who love to run. I had trouble imagining this when I was starting out, back when I couldn't haul myself around a single lap without feeling like I was going to suck my lungs inside out. But as my cardiovascular fitness improved and my heart and lungs became stronger, I began to find running very satisfying. It went from being painful, to being challenging, to finally being fairly easy. These days I actually enjoy it, and I know many other runners who would say the same thing. I am also back to playing tennis, with *no* knee pain!

Another thing I realized is that I love to lift weights. It not only strengthens me physically, but mentally as well. If you do it correctly and lift weights that are heavy enough to challenge and change you it's hard work, and I've learned that it should never stop being somewhat difficult. That's how you improve and grow. While Renita has introduced me to routines that are more interesting than lifting on those machines used by sweaty guys at the gym, it's never going to be as fun as, say, skiing or playing tennis. But when you weigh the benefits, you can't deny that it's well worth every drop of sweat. It's not just a matter of being able to swing across the playground equipment with ease, it's a matter of being able to lift yourself out of a chair as you approach old age. The nasty little secret of modern medicine is that doctors can and often do keep us alive for years past the time when we can enjoy ourselves because we haven't kept our muscles and joints in good condition. You can sit back now and just let time take its toll, or you can meet it head on.

When I made the decision to contact Renita it was about my weight. But as I've improved my fitness level I've noticed something important: all of those aches and pains that I thought were just a part of getting older no longer plague me. My back no longer aches when I get up in the morning. My knees don't hurt. I do sometimes have sore muscles and the occasional twinge from a tough workout, but that feels like progress rather than old age.

It's also improved my mental sharpness, and that makes sense. Science is now proving that a diet rich in antioxidants along with regular exercise can delay or even ward off Alzheimer's disease and other forms of dementia. Studies done at the Alzheimer's Research Center appear to show that a daily brisk walk can, by itself, cut your risk by 45 percent because the increased movement pumps more blood and oxygen to your brain. It also triggers your body to secrete chemicals that protect the brain and can actually encourage the growth of neurons. Even if you were predisposed to Alzheimer's disease, regular medium intensity exercise can ward it off long enough that you never experience the symptoms during your lifetime. And all of that isn't taking into account the protective potential that could ward off a whole host of other health disasters such as cardiovascular disease, diabetes, and cancer.

Another added bonus: strength training and cardio workouts have cut my stress level in half. When I'm really irritated by someone or something I can take that fight-or-flight response that goes with anger and put it toward a tough workout. By the time I'm finished I always feel better, and it helps me sleep. I'm not just imagining this, either. Researchers at the Mayo Clinic say exercise boosts your endorphin levels, which improves your mood. It allows you to focus on your body and its movements rather than your problems, which gives you a bit of a vacation from whatever's bugging you. And it does, indeed, improve your ability to sleep, which in itself helps you deal with stress. There are so many reasons to do it that it only makes sense to get started.

If you're clever about it, you can sneak weight lifting into your daily routine. When my daughter was a baby she was only happy if I carried her. My arms were in great shape because for a year I carried around a steadily increasing amount of weight, shifting the baby from arm to arm. So lift your baby over your head, do squats while you're cooking dinner, do step-ups the next time you have to climb the stairs to put away the laundry. Or you can stop what you're doing right now and go swing a kettle bell. The point is, get up!

Activity has always come easy for me. I love to work and I love to work out. I was born that way, raised that way, and it definitely is my sweet spot. I love productivity. To set a goal, do the work, and blow the goal out of the water gets me fired up! I found that God gave me this strength of exercise and movement to inspire others to get up and get moving! Remember, we are always given a strength to share with others. It comes easily and naturally for me. As a result, I have acquired over 25 health and fitness certifications. I love to teach everything from Pilates to kickboxing! I currently lead all ages, from children to people in their 90s to a healthier life. From pregnant moms to athletes, I love making a difference! Health is making a choice that you want to be well and you are willing to do something about that choice! Choosing to change happens in a moment. The change itself happens over time.

There comes a point where we need to quit thinking about it and praying about it, and get to work! Sometimes people feel like they need to know everything before they start exercising, but I have found that over-analysis leads to paralysis. Action produces more action and inactivity leads to more lethargy, pain, and often, depression. An active lifestyle produces incredible results in body, soul, and spirit. Studies show that when individuals work out for at least 20 minutes, six days a

week, their hormone levels improve, which minimizes the risk of depression. I have created two online programs to help your journey! They are both incredible, affordable, and fun! Join www.millionstepchallenge.com or www.allstrongmoms.com. I have seen incredible results with people who join these online workout programs. People in their 70s who are getting in the best shape of their lives! Moms who are getting their bodies back after six children. Women who couldn't walk without huffing and puffing are now running three times a week. Once they start, I find people marching in place while washing the dishes, doing knee lifts while waiting in line at the grocery store, taking the stairs, and parking at the last spot in the lot. All of those little decisions lead to big results. There definitely is such a thing as an "active lifestyle."

If you haven't exercised in decades, walking is the place to start. Start by walking around your block daily. On the first week, do it once. On the second week, walk around the block two times. Before long, you'll be doing it four times, and that's the equivalent of one mile!

I also love tracking devices such as Fitbit, Jawbone, or even an old-fashioned pedometer. It is important to know where you are so you know where you are going. A goal gives us a focal point to shoot for.

Begin by answering the question *why*? Why do you want this? Think big! How will making these healthy changes affect your destiny? Your legacy?

On this question, go deep emotionally to discover the real reason you want to lose weight. What do you want to gain by getting healthy?

Now set a SMART CPR goal.

- S- specific
- M- measurable
- A- activity oriented
- R- realistic
- T- timed
- C- celebrate
- P- positive
- R- read your goals out loud

Be specific with it. The clearer you are on your goal, the more likely you are to achieve it.

_____

_____

Make it measurable. Decide how you are going to track progress. Examples would be to measure yourself, weigh yourself, or use an activity tracking device.

_____

_____

Become activity oriented. Decide what daily activities you will be doing to reach your goal.

_____

_____

Be realistic, setting goals that are challenging, yet attainable.

_____

_____

Your goals should be timed, which means every goal should have a start date and a date by which you hope to meet your goal, although you can always adjust the end date. Remember the only way you won't reach your goal is by quitting.

_____

_____

Celebrate your victories along the way. Find ways to reward yourself that don't involve food.

_____

_____

Be positive. Write three positive health decisions daily. Make sure what you are telling yourself is affirming. In fact, also write three positive things you have already accomplished for your health.

_____

_____

Read your goals out loud. Studies show people who read their goals out loud three times per day are more likely to reach them. When will you read your goals and where will they be posted? Mine are on my bathroom mirror in red lipstick.

_____

_____

Now that you know where you want to go, let's talk about some specific ways to incorporate fitness training into your daily life. First, some things to keep in mind.

The lean muscle on your body acts like a fireplace for your metabolism. If you want that fire roaring, it is important to maintain and develop as much lean muscle as possible. As you age, you naturally lose about 7% of lean muscle each decade after the age of 25. If you are not doing something with exercise and strength training to combat that, you will most likely feel like Gumby or the Pillsbury Dough Boy. Your lean muscle also protects your bones, so weight bearing activity is crucial to prevention of osteoporosis. Think strong and healthy, not skinny and flabby. The more muscle tissue you can activate during each workout, the faster your metabolism will become. You should strength train a minimum of two to three times per week, and remember your muscle tissue starts to atrophy after about 72 hours of not working it.

Which exercise is the best? After 20 years in health and fitness, I know what produces results. As I told you earlier, nutrition will account for 80% of your weight loss, and will safeguard your overall health. The same goes for developing lean muscle. Again, nutrition is the key, and complete protein is crucial.

The balance of PFC Every 3 approximately 30 to 45 minutes before a workout will maximize your results! Make sure you always eat before your workout. It stabilizes your blood sugar and allows your body to release stored fat so your muscles can burn it up as fuel.

Which exercises burn the most fat?

1. Strength training with weights or kettlebells
    • You will burn fat for up to 36 hours after a strength training workout.
2. Body Weight Strength Training
    • You will also burn fat for up to 36 hours and it's super effective for people with no equipment or for those just beginning.
3. HIIT (High Intensity Interval Training)
    • Phenomenal workout for people who only have 20 minutes and want to maximize their time. This

combines strength and cardio and results occur quickly. You will continue to burn fat for up to three hours after a HIIT workout.

- If you combine HIIT with strength training you again will burn fat for up to 36 hours. This is one of my favorite ways to exercise!

4. Cardiovascular Exercise
   - Great place to start if it's been a while since you worked out. Also a phenomenal low impact activity. It may take a bit longer to see results, but the internal conditioning is excellent. If you have extra time, cardiovascular activities like walking or riding bike are excellent ways to condition your body and burn fat. It will take more of this type of activity than HIIT to see results. But, hey, we have the rest of our lives to get healthy, so let's go!

5. Balance and Flexibility
   - Do balance exercises daily. They help with core strength and coordination as you age. It can be as simple as standing on one leg while washing dishes.

Flexibility increases fastest if you do it at least three times per week. I recommend doing stretching exercises after every workout, because the muscle is warm and will naturally be more pliable. Only stretch a warm muscle. Think of it like taffy. Imagine trying to stretch cold taffy. Now imagine trying to stretch warm taffy. It's much more effective to stretch and lengthen a warmed-up muscle (dynamic stretching). Do dynamic stretches during the warm up and static stretches during the cool down! (A static stretch is stationary. You generally hold the stretch for 20 seconds or longer.)

For examples of great workouts you can do daily, go to www.millionstepchallenge.com or www.allstrongmoms.com.

Within 20 minutes after a workout, consume a complete protein source, which will help you to rebuild your muscles. Eggs or tuna (P and F), and some fruit (C), would be a great combo.

POWER VERSE:

Then the Lord replied, "Write down the revelation and make it plain on tablets, so that a herald may run with it." -Habakkuk 2:2 NIV

Chapter 24
Race Day!

"Let him run Ronnie, let him run!"- *Secretariat*

If you ever have a serious asthma attack, you'll never forget it. It's a very scary feeling. I have always equated running with the feeling that I can't breathe, and that feeling was enough to make me vow to avoid distance running at all costs.

When Renita and I started training, things went well at first aside from a case of shin splints which resolved fairly quickly. But about six weeks before the race, and before I was able to complete an entire 5K, I picked up a flu virus that brought with it a fever, fatigue, laryngitis, a severe sore throat and a cough. Renita was showing up at my house with hot soup and eucalyptus salts for my bath, along with a variety of other natural remedies to go with the meds the doctor prescribed, but it was not a fast-moving illness. The fever subsided after about a week, but the cough just wouldn't give up, despite treatment with inhaled corticosteroids. In other words, the asthma was back, especially when I tried to run.

I'm fairly competitive and I wasn't ready to give up on the race idea. For one thing, I'd advertised it and we'd made such a big deal about it that I thought if I were to cancel, it would feel like defeat and would be embarrassing. And even though common sense told me the viewers would understand illness, I kept postponing the moment when I'd have to pull the plug. I'm not sure, but I suspect that Renita was preparing to find another race a little later in the summer. Still, she was never anything but positive and upbeat. I don't believe I've ever met a more encouraging person. When I couldn't run, we walked. One day we were scoping out the course for the race we'd chosen and I was clearly struggling just walking, so we stopped and did strength training at a nearby picnic area instead. I got really tired of being sick and was just a tad mopey. Okay, more than a tad. But she'd always show up with a big smile and find some inspiring thing to say and after visiting with her I always felt better. That's a rare quality, and one I greatly admire.

Perhaps it was her positive reinforcement, perhaps it was nature just taking its course, but I slowly started to improve as race day approached and we again hit the track, although I was running with my inhaler in my hand. My times had slowed and I actually felt like I was going backwards. Three weeks before the race I made it two miles without stopping. Two weeks prior, it was two and a half miles. The goal wasn't to get a great time. Rather, it was to go as far as possible without having to take a break. I didn't run three miles until two days prior to race day, and it wasn't until the day before that I finally felt like I could take a deep breath without using my inhaler first. I truly did improve just in the nick of time, but it remained to be seen whether I could make it the entire 5 kilometers.

The race itself would have been fun if I hadn't been so nervous. I was terrified that I wouldn't be able to run the whole thing. I'm not sure why it was such a big deal. To add to the fun, and to offer encouragement, my husband and daughter also signed up to run, and so did Renita's entire family. They all disappeared into the pack ahead of us, but Renita stayed with me the whole way. What made it particularly challenging was the fact that the course wasn't marked, so we had no idea how far we'd come. It was a color splash event and I knew that there were five color stations, so the only real indication we had of the distance from the finish line was to count the stations.

As we were running, Renita was chatting and greeting people and talking to me to distract me. She kept up a running dialogue. I suppose we were about halfway through when she looked over at me and said, "You aren't saying much. Are you okay?" I just nodded. Truthfully, I didn't have enough breath to talk. I just kept putting one foot in front of the other and eventually I saw the finish line in the distance. That was a big moment! Cliff and Meghanne were standing right there with a bottle of water and big hugs. You'd have thought it was a marathon. But let's be honest, finishing that race was a big accomplishment for me! I felt just the way I'd felt years earlier climbing that mountain because (I can say it now) I was just as scared.

A major opportunity for me to assist Monica in the completion of her 5K was not only to train her physically, but to help her captivate her thoughts and beliefs and get them headed toward victory. She carried the inhaler during our first few weeks of training. I helped her to take control of her respirations by thinking about them. With each stride, her breathing got stronger. We would count 1,2,3,4, inhale, 1,2,3,4, exhale. I taught her that by focusing on your breath and elongating it instead of letting it get shorter and shorter, which eventually makes you feel like you are going to hyperventilate, you can slow down your rate of respiration. Some people let their breath control them which makes them panic, and others control their breath.

I realized over the years of training clients that you can get control of your breath by getting control of your thoughts, and vice versa. When your mind is scared, your respiration increases. My job was to help Monica focus her thoughts on each step and coordinating her breath. As a result, her lung capacity strengthened, especially as it was coupled with good nutrition

and plenty of water. Thank God she had quit drinking Diet Coke, as that dehydrates our bodies. Studies now show a person's asthma and allergies can be greatly minimized just by being well hydrated.

After week three, Monica left her inhaler in the car. I didn't see it again until she got the nasty virus a month before the race. But then again, the race was getting closer. Much of training is overcoming the beliefs we have about ourselves. Remember, Monica had quit track and field in her youth due to breathing. I was going to help her make sure that it wasn't going to happen again.

Sometimes, if you spend enough time with someone who believes in you, then you'll start to believe too. I know this is a faith journey. Fear and faith do not go hand in hand. Where fear exists, faith cannot. Since I love the Lord with all my heart and believe His plans for me are amazing, I stand on that truth. I know Monica has strong faith in God as well, so sticking with her to encourage her to keep running the race was easy. For no longer than a few seconds did I feel like we were going to reschedule that race. I read a book once that said whatever you focus on becomes your reality. We were focusing on running that race! Monica had trained appropriately and has a strong mental fortitude. The training may have simmered a bit when she got hit a few times with crazy symptoms, but we just kept forging on, never skipping a workout. We just modified it at times so we wouldn't break her down, but instead, strengthen her (even if the inhaler was sitting on the elliptical). The foundational changes we had made with her nutrition, cardio and strength training were lifting her up through this challenging finale.

Monica finished the Color Run right beside me. As it says in Ecclesiastes 4:9, "Two people are better than one, for they can help each other succeed." Cliff and their daughter stood at the finish line to embrace her! She didn't have to use her inhaler during the run, either. As we ran the race, everyone along the path encouraged Monica by saying how watching her on TV had inspired them to get healthy and get moving. I am convinced that had she not done the race it would have been caving in to fear. It was the dirty devil's plan to have her not run that day. "The thief comes only to steal and kill and destroy; I have come that they may have life, and have it to the full." – John 10:10. We chose faith on race day, and God always multiplies our efforts. I witnessed it that day as hundreds encouraged her and were encouraged by her. It allowed people to believe in themselves, and think that if Monica did it, they could too! No matter where they were on their health journey, she inspired so many to get up and go for it!

Everyone has something they are dealing with when it comes to health. Whether it is an injury, or an individual just beginning with bad knees, everyone could have an excuse to not exercise. When Monica started she had an achy knee that we were respectful of. Now, I never hear her mention that knee. She is walking and running three times a week! She plays tennis twice a week! She strength trains 2-3 times a week! In addition, she bought a heart rate monitor and a Jawbone tracking device and continues to get over 10,000 steps a day! She completed her millions steps in 90 days at www.millionstepchallenge.com and is now rocking the workouts at www.allstrongmoms.com. She is a strong mom! In fact over 1,500 people have completed the million step challenge with Monica and over 2,500 moms are now part of ALL STRONG MOMS!

Monica is definitely healthy! She probably would have been a state track athlete in her youth. Thank God she regained her youthfulness and is running the race set before her now! That race is called LIFE!

Now… Are you ready to GET UP AND GO FOR IT?

POWER VERSE:

"Therefore, since we are surrounded by such a great cloud of witnesses, let us throw off everything that hinders and the sin that so easily entangles. And let us run with perseverance the race marked out for us, fixing our eyes on Jesus, the pioneer and perfecter of our faith." -Hebrews 12:1-2 NIV

Nice and F.A.T.

If you are tired of being F.A.T. and are ready to receive a 7 day FREE Zen PFC detox meal plan, text FAT to 57711. This will help you stay connected with Renita and Monica.

You may receive up to 4 messages per week. Message and data rates may apply when sending & receiving text messages. Msgs sent from automated system. Consent not required to purchase goods/services. Text STOP to 57711 to opt-out. Text HELP to 57711 for assistance or call 800-211-2001. To view our Privacy Policy, please visit www.sentextsolutions.com/privacypolicy.

ABOUT THE AUTHORS

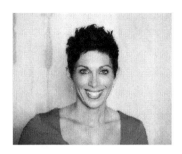

Renita Brannan is a global health professional with over 20 years of experience. She is a Certified Biblical Health Coach, ACE Certified Advanced Personal Trainer, Group Fitness Instructor, and Lifestyle & Weight Management Consultant. Renita is also a Certified Venice Nutrition Coach who was recently featured on CNN HLN for helping North Dakota lose over 50,000 lbs of fat. She is a Jeunesse entrepreneur in which she teaches PFC every 3 globally. She is co-creator of www.allstrongmoms.com and www.pfcplate.com where she empowers individuals to nourish their bodies to achieve amazing health. Renita resides in Bismarck, ND with her husband Scott, three healthy boys Beau, Truitt, and Rocco, as well as her dog, Zoe.

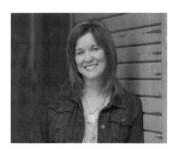

Monica Hannan is a three-time Emmy-award-winning news manager and anchor for KFYR-TV. She has also authored the books *Gift of Death – A Message of Comfort of Hope* and *The Dream Maker.* Her articles on history, travel and health have appeared in regional and national magazines.

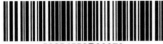

59254553R00070

Made in the USA
Lexington, KY
29 December 2016